FAITH THROUGH CANCER

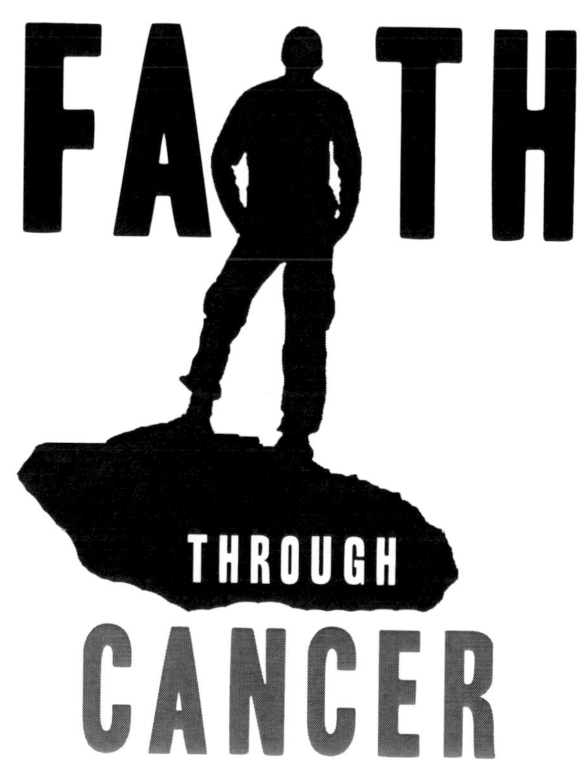

A HUSBAND'S HOPE FOR HEALING

BOB HOWE

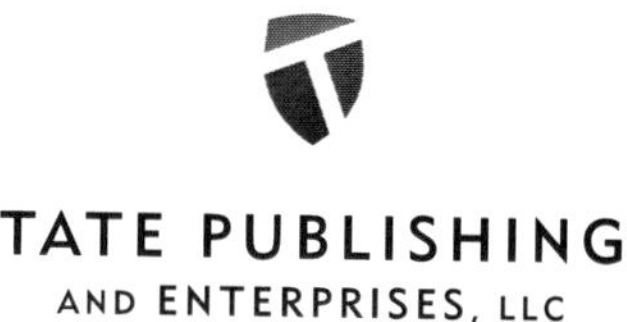

TATE PUBLISHING
AND ENTERPRISES, LLC

Published by Tate Publishing & Enterprises, LLC
127 E. Trade Center Terrace | Mustang, Oklahoma 73064 USA
1.888.361.9473 | www.tatepublishing.com

Tate Publishing is committed to excellence in the publishing industry. The company reflects the philosophy established by the founders, based on Psalm 68:11,
"The Lord gave the word and great was the company of those who published it."

Cover design by Lucia Renz
Interior design by Chelsea Womble

Published in the United States of America

ISBN: 978-1-61862-855-8
1. Biography & Autobiography / Personal Memoirs
2. Health & Fitness / Diseases / Cancer
12.05.02

DEDICATION

To my wife: I know for sure that cancer is a terrible and painful disease, and I regret that you had to go through it. Cancer has taught me more about Christ and what is truly important. It has given me a greater love for you, our family, and of course Jesus Christ.

TABLE OF CONTENTS

THE CRISIS BEGINS

"Why don't you call your doctor?" I said. "He has had more than enough time to look at that report."

Linda had been lying sick on the sofa or in the bed for nearly two months now. No actual problems had been found, and treatments for possible problems the doctors thought she might have had not been successful. We had been praying, but we didn't even know what to pray about.

Linda said, "Okay, I will call."

I think we had both been worried about this report. She kept saying she felt better, but I could see she didn't. I was afraid there would still be no answers and more expensive tests to take. Of course, one of my thoughts was, *How are we going to pay for this?*

I am self employed and work had almost stopped. We did not have health insurance at that time because of the lack of work. It was not a good time for any kind of sickness to come into our lives, but there never is a good time.

It was truly amazing how God worked. I was greatly confused through all of this in the beginning, wondering what God was going to do to make things work out. I knew He was there, I knew He cared, but we had been spiraling downhill for some time, in work and in Linda's health. I have learned over the years that God never answers the way my feeble little mind thinks He should. He answers in amazing ways that I would never have thought of.

My wife and I are in our late fifties. I was saved when I was twelve, but never really turned to God until my late thirties. Linda and my kids were always praying for me to live for Christ and it took a while for me to open my eyes. At this point we were just praying for a positive report on the CAT scan. We believed our hope and our faith would produce a good outcome. What could go wrong with God on our side?

Linda explained to the nurse on the phone who she was and what she had called for. After a few minutes of discussion, the nurse informed her that the doctor would call back as soon as he could.

"I'd hoped they would have some answers today," I said in disappointment. "I hate to wait through another weekend. I just want to know what to ask God."

"Be patient, they will call," Linda replied.

I just rolled my eyes and fell back into my chair.

"They have a pill for everything except patience," I said. "I know nothing will happen today. I just want to know what is wrong. I am tired of you being sick and not knowing why."

We had seen many miracles and wonders from our past, but most of them belonged to someone else. Oh yes, we had some blessings of our own, but we quickly forgot them when things were good. It was often easier to see the blessings when they were over, than it was when we were walking through them. We were about to encounter another part of our lives where Jesus had to carry us, but we didn't know it yet.

Only ten minutes had passed and the phone rang. The caller ID said it was the doctor's office. *That,* I thought, *was a blessing.* I didn't expect a response so soon.

I got up and handed the cordless phone to Linda. After thirty-three years of marriage, I had learned how to read my wife's thoughts in her face. I could not hear the doctor, but I could tell Linda was not hearing what she wanted to hear. Why do we always think the worst? That's just what I did. *Is something taking her life? How could I go on without her?* We had talked about death in our past, but it never seemed more real than it did at that time. I thought w*e could get more tests because this doctor might be wrong. Bad things couldn't come our way; we belong to God and why would I possibly think about death?* But inside I knew it was a big problem of some kind because Linda had been sick far too long.

Linda was on the phone for another ten minutes as I grew more and more impatient. Finally, she hung up and turned to look at me. Without a word she began to cry. I sat down beside her and cried with her. I knew our lives would be changed in ways we never wanted to talk about. I was afraid for her and terrified for myself. She hadn't said what it was, but I knew it wasn't going to be good. Part of me wanted to know what it was, but most of me just wanted it to go away.

I told her, "God has always been here for us, and you know He is here now."

"I have cancer," she said, and we cried even more.

We prayed the best we could through the tears. We knew all the Bible verses. God is the healer (Exodus 15:26). Believers will pray and heal the sick (Mark 16:17-18). Ask and you shall receive (Luke 11:9). Where two of you gather, ask anything and our Father will do it for you (Matthew 18:19). Believe you have received what you have asked, and it will be yours (Mark 11:24).

We also knew cancer could kill. We knew some survive. Both were hard to consider when they didn't exist in our life five minutes ago.

"I have a grandchild on the way," Linda said. "I want to hold her."

"You will."

"I want to be with all of my grandchildren to see them grow up. I want to live."

"You will live. God isn't done with you yet. And you know I can't do without you. Who would feed me?"

Jokes are not always the best approach, but I didn't know what to say. I'm not sure which of us was feeling worse. Linda might have cancer, and the emotional ride was not helping either of us.

It seemed like only a few minutes had passed when the phone rang again. *But wait*, I thought, we didn't want to talk to anyone else right then. We were still wrestling with the new emotions that had just found us during the last phone call. *What if it is one of our kids? We weren't ready to tell them.* I checked the caller ID, and it was the doctor's office again. *Maybe our prayers have already worked! Maybe the doctor gave us the wrong report! Maybe we can go back to a normal life!*

I quickly handed the phone to Linda and watched her as she talked.

"Okay. Okay," she said. "That is only thirty minutes from now."

I thought I could see a spark of hope through her tears and in her voice. Perhaps an error was found and our prayers had been answered. *Maybe there is no cancer, and we can forget this ever happened.*

"We will leave right now and get there as soon as we can," she said as she hung up the phone.

"Where are we going? What did the doctor say?"

We were still in our pajamas.

"Get dressed," she said. "We have an appointment with the Cancer Care Center in thirty minutes. My doctor got me in to see one of the best doctors in the state."

"That's great! Maybe he could see that this is all a mistake."

Our time for weeping was cut short. So was our time to get across town. We knew we would be at least twenty minutes late, but hoped the doctor would still see us. On the way, we talked about our kids. How would we tell them if there was cancer? Where would the money come from even for minor medical needs? But we talked about God even more. How do people face problems like this if they don't know Jesus? How should we act when we face these problems? In our rush to get to our destination, the tears briefly stopped. Later, we would have more time to reflect on the day's events.

We arrived thirty minutes late. I dropped Linda off at the glass front doors so she could sit and wait for me to park the car. She was not strong enough for the long walk from the parking lot. I parked the car and ran back to the building. We entered the foyer that was filled with plants and trees, and had a pond in the center surrounded by a rock walkway. There was a waterfall that drew our attention to the brass park benches nearby. Maybe later we could sit there and talk.

We found the doors to the Cancer Care Center on the second floor. It was a strange feeling walking through the doors of a place it seemed we didn't belong. There were people both young and old, some without hair and some in wheel chairs.

I informed the receptionist behind the desk who we were, and we took a seat. The place was like most doctors' offices, lots of seats full of people looking at their cell phones or reading a magazine. A small television was up in the corner with no one paying any attention to it.

I whispered to my wife, "God is here with us."

I don't know if she heard me or not. I think she was busy talking to God.

It was only a few minutes before they called for Linda to come back to the admission office. We spent the next two and a half hours going over payment methods, family history, work status, current medications, and other information. Most of the questions were easy enough, but we still had no idea how to pay for it. They gave us a list of people and places to call next week to help us find the answers we desperately needed. Then it was back to the waiting room again.

We wondered when they might see us. Do they not know how important our situation is? Doesn't the Cancer Center know Linda might have cancer? It is truly amazing how our minds operate when we are in a stressful situation. It is truly amazing how my mind would focus on the worse thoughts instead of the good in this stressful situation.

The Bible tells us in 1 Peter 5:7 to give all our worries and anxiety to Christ. I find it hard to let go of mine sometimes. I don't want them, but maybe I need to hold them for a while before I give them up to Christ. How else could we know the good God has for us if we never knew the bad? I just wanted to take Linda home and never hear the word cancer again.

At 4:45 p.m., Linda was called to see the doctor. We went in together. It was the usual small room with two chairs, a desk with a sink, and an examination table. I studied the charts on the wall and Linda sat down and closed her eyes.

In a short time the doctor entered the room. He was very tall and most of his hair was gray, but he was younger than Linda and I. *This is good* I thought, *not too old, not too young*. We talked for a while, and I was asked to leave the room for the examination, so I left to find my way back to the waiting room.

As I searched for the room, I still did not believe the reports. *How could Linda have cancer? How would we tell the kids?* I was confused. *How could this happen to us?*

I entered the waiting room and found a seat. I thought, *if she does have cancer, I'd better get used to this waiting*. But waiting is not something I am very good at. I have the Bible on my Blackberry so I sat down and opened it to read. I read for almost an hour before I realized I could not remember what I had just read. I wasn't really reading; I was still astonished by the day. I closed my phone and realized I didn't even know what book of the Bible I had been looking at.

Ten more minutes passed as I sat there in a daze, and then I was called back to the room where I had left Linda. We were told that she had ovarian cancer.

"If you have to have cancer," Dr. Kevin said, "this is the best cancer to have. We have great success at beating this one."

I never thought about one cancer being better than another. How could we feel good about having the best cancer when we didn't want any at all? Dr. Kevin told us many things that hour, almost too much to take in. It was Friday, March 20, and he scheduled the surgery for April first. He tried to schedule the surgery for the next week, but he could not get her in that soon. The immediate priority Dr. Kevin was placing on the surgery made us feel it was very critical. He explained to us the size of the tumor and its location. He told us the tumor had overtaken the ovaries and the uterus and that they would have to be removed. It all seemed so normal to him, but we had a million thoughts and a million uncertainties. His words became like the Bible I was just reading. I could not understand his words, and I didn't want to hear them. I was still living and acting like this couldn't be for us.

"The operation usually takes place in about two or three hours," Dr. Kevin said. "But if it should take a little longer, don't let that worry you. It's not necessarily a bad thing. We can't see the entire tumor until we get inside."

As you might imagine, this was not making us feel any better, especially since earlier that day, I thought nothing much would happen. Boy, was I wrong. I vaguely remembered hearing the word *surgery* as I tried to process all of this.

"What happens after surgery?" I asked.

He said, "Linda will need to go through chemotherapy treatments. We will talk about that after the surgery, but remember that chemo treatments today are not the same as they were in your grandmother's day."

I wasn't sure what that was supposed to mean, but the doctor and all of his staff were very good at trying to erase our fears. I wasn't so sure it made us feel any better. They were all so full of confidence and so sure of what was going on. We got the feeling that only good things could happen here, but I was still in my own dreamland. We must have seen and talked to ten people that day, all of them filling us with more information than we could contain. There was a lot to think about, and we were both glad when it was time to go home.

Dr. Kevin finished with us, and we left his office. Our day had been greatly changed from what it was when we woke up that morning. Cancer? Surgery in two weeks? How would this change the next few months or the next few years? We had the weekend to think and pray about all that had happened, and now we knew what to pray about.

God can cure cancer in two weeks, I thought. *God could cure cancer in one day.* We were still holding onto that hope.

We didn't talk much as I walked Linda to the entrance doors. We were both deep in our own thoughts. She waited in silence on the park bench as I went to get the car. I pulled up to the glass doors and helped Linda into the car.

"I have to go tell the kids," Linda said after she got in.

"Tonight? It's been a long day. Why don't you wait until tomorrow?"

"No, I have to tell them now, and not on the phone," she said.

She wanted to go to Wendy's house first. She is the oldest. I called ahead to make sure she was home. It would be close to bedtime for her kids, so I was sure she would be home, and she was.

Both of our kids knew we were waiting on the CAT scan report this week, so when we showed up, Wendy knew we had some important news. We told her of the day's events as she tended to her children in the front room, getting them ready for bed. I watched her as she worked, thinking how blessed Linda and I were, because we didn't have to do that anymore. Grandkids were great to play with for a while, and then we could send them home again.

Linda and Wendy continued to talk as they took the kids to their rooms. I stayed in the front room thinking how much better Wendy received the news than I did. It is hard for me to tell at times with Wendy because she can hide her real emotions so well. Her expression did not appear to change as mine did, but her mother would know. Her husband was working late, and I knew Linda needed to rest, so we weren't going to stay long. They could talk more tomorrow on the phone.

While they were talking, I called ahead to my other daughter's house. Leslie was home, and I informed her we would be coming over shortly for a visit about our day at the doctor's office. Big mistake on my part; I should have gone over without calling.

When we got to her house she was finishing with putting her daughter to bed. Linda and Leslie spent the next few minutes in the bedroom hugging and kissing our granddaughter. Leslie's husband, Derek, and I talked in the front room.

"Leslie was worried and crying after you called," he said. "She is afraid her mom might be dying or something."

"I didn't tell her anything," I said. "Maybe I should not have called ahead."

I sometimes forget she is so sensitive. The fact that I called instead of her mother was enough to set off an alarm. I paused in thought for a moment, giving thanks to God for two of the best sons-in-law a father could have. I knew they would both take good care of their wives, and I thanked God they found each other.

"Leslie has been worried all week waiting for the test results," he said. "Did they find anything?"

"Yeah, we have been worried too."

Linda and Leslie came back into the front room. We all sat down, and Linda and I explained our day to them the best we could. Leslie was happy to know what was going on instead of wondering like we had been doing. No one was happy about the cancer, but we finally had a small amount of relief in knowing a solution was in progress. We prayed for a quick solution, and I took Linda home to rest. They too would talk more tomorrow.

We passed on the information we received that day to our church and a few other churches. We now knew what to ask of God, and we quickly began seeing the hand of God in motion. Our church family and out daughters' church families said many prayers that weekend and for many weeks following.

It was good to return home to our own furniture and to a familiar place where we felt safe. The day kept us busy and kept our minds from working on our worst thoughts. God knew we needed to be active and moving around that day instead of waiting until next week.

"You know, God is not done with us yet," I said.

"I know."

"The kids took the news pretty well."

"They had to know today."

Linda had a kidney disease when she was twelve. Back then, there was no cure, but the family told me she was healed by God's hand and much prayer from Grandma. I didn't meet Linda until we were twenty, and without Grandma's prayers I might not have gotten to know her at all.

"God healed you when you were twelve so you would be around to help me find my way," I said. "He will heal you again. I still need you."

"I never thought I would have cancer."

"It's not your cancer. Satan is the father of cancer, and we're giving it back."

"Why couldn't it have been something easier?"

"Satan doesn't want it to be easy. He wants you to give up."

"I have too much to live for."

"God never gives us more than we can handle, and I know He will help us through this."

"But I don't want to do this."

I took her in my arms, and we sat in silence for a long time. We were unsure of the journey ahead of us, but we were together that night as we had always been and we knew that would not change. We knew we had each other, and we knew God was on our side.

We spent the rest of the evening sharing our thoughts with each other and with God. I can't even imagine how people can walk the road we were about to take without Jesus Christ in their lives. That day we received a blow from Satan, and he doesn't give up easy. There was more to come. We know God knows how to rescue us from our trials. It was time for us to put on all the armor of God (Eph. 6:11), and we did this with great confidence in our time of need.

The blessings and the crisis from that one day were already working on pulling the family closer together. Without any work on our part, God put us in the hands of one of the best surgeons in Oklahoma. He gave us some answers on the same day that we became aware of the problem, and He gave us the weekend to gather our thoughts to face the problems of the weeks that lie ahead.

We thanked God that He is with us and for the gifts of this day (Phil. 4:6 NLT). *Thank you, Jesus, for all you have done.*

FINANCES

We spent a lot of time on the phone that Saturday, informing friends and family about Linda's condition. On Sunday, our Sunday school class at church provided much love and prayers. We received plenty of hugs and volunteers to help with whatever we needed. We were unable to stay for all the services of the day as Linda was worn out, so we returned home for the rest of the day.

When Monday morning arrived, it was time to begin the next challenge that lay ahead. Our first step was to find some way to help to pay for this. One of our greatest fears was wondering if the hospitals would work with us without insurance. The Cancer Care Center gave us a list of places to contact for help. The first stop was the Department of Human Services. This was difficult because we had never needed to ask for help from anyone except for small problems for a day or two, and that help was from friends. I had always taken care of my family and needed help from no one, but I knew I needed help with this expense. No one can afford the medical expense like we had ahead of us without insurance, and we were without it. DHS is the place where people in need of food stamps, people in need of housing, people with great medical problems come, and on this day, we were those people.

We packed a bag with sandwiches and a few snacks to take with us. We did not want to be out eating lunch if they called our name. It was hard for Linda to sit up for an hour at a time, and we knew a government office would be an all-day event.

We drove downtown, and I parked as close as I could so Linda would not have to walk far. This was not an attractive part of town, and I was afraid to drop her off at the door. There were many people coming in and going out of the building, and some of them were not very happy. We knew we had to come to this place, but we had not been looking forward to it. Jesus said not to worry about anything, but it was hard to do when we were standing in scary places. Don't worry about tomorrow; today's trouble is enough for today (Matt. 6:34). We had no idea what was inside of DHS, but it made us a little fearful. It wasn't just the bad part of town we were in, but what we might find out when we got inside that made us anxious. We hoped and prayed we could get some help.

We entered through a double door into a short hallway. Then a revolving door led to the metal detector and the policemen. We emptied our pockets and our bags into a tray and passed through an x-ray machine. We stepped through the metal detector and picked up our things on the other side. We had the same feeling we'd had at the Cancer Care Center. *We don't belong here. This is not the way we live.* We were truly feeling lost, but God said He would never leave us (Heb.13:5).

DHS has four floors for the people coming in seeking help. We had no idea where to go, so we started on floor one. There had to be over a hundred people in that lobby. It was a bit frightening because so many people were there that came from a different lifestyle than our own. Some of them looked homeless, some had physical disabilities, and some had very strange-looking clothes. I know God looks at the heart and not what you and I see on the outside (Heb. 4:12). I'm glad He does, because I was sure my appearance also looked strange to some of the people in that place.

I said a short, silent prayer for the people in that room that they might all find their needs met here. Then I saw a sign that said, "Apply here for food stamps. Take a number."

"I think this is the wrong floor," I told my wife.

I sure hoped it was the wrong floor. "Take a number" with that many people would mean the rest of the day for sure. We went back to the elevator to explore the second floor.

As soon as the doors opened, I saw a sign that said "Medical Assistance." The area had a small lobby with only a few people. I thought, *This is great. The Lord is surely with us.* We walked forward to talk to the receptionist behind the glass wall.

I told her, "My wife is having surgery in a few days, and we need to see someone for some medical help."

"Do you have an appointment?"

She was a big woman and didn't look like she took any attitude from anyone. I was sure she was flooded with such people in this job.

"No," I said. "Our doctor told us to come up here."

"You will have to go down to the first floor."

I noticed, even though she looked rough, that she had a lot of Christian items around her desk. Maybe that was to keep her from going crazy around so many mixed-up people.

I said with my best possible Christian spirit, "I just came from there. The sign said food stamps. We are not looking for food stamps. We have never been here before. Can you help us find the place to get medical assistance?"

She looked at me for the first time, smiled, and said, "Are you needing Medicaid?"

"I think so. Will that help with my wife's surgery?"

"Yes," she said as she handed me some papers. "Fill these out and bring them back to me."

"Thank you," I said with a smile.

We sat down to fill out the papers. I did most of the writing, because it was a struggle for Linda. There were about nine pages to be filled out. We brought last year's tax returns and other information with us. The Cancer Center warned us we would need them. We were afraid that if we forgot something, it might add another day to getting some help so we brought more information with us than we needed. Linda could not take many days of this.

In a short time, I took the papers back to the receptionist and asked, "Do you know how long it might be before we can see someone? My wife is very tired from the cancer."

I thought if she knew about the cancer it might speed things up.

"They will send you a report in about three weeks," she said.

"Three weeks! But she has surgery in a few days! Can we see someone today?"

She smiled at us again in a way that would not reveal her soft heart in this rough environment. I think she realized we were truly in a new world and didn't know what we were doing.

She explained to us that they would send a letter in about three weeks that would tell us that our request had been denied. "Don't worry about that," she said. "That is standard procedure. Call the number on the page to ask for an interview. You also need to call the Social Security office and talk to them. Each of these calls will give you further directions on what you need to do. You have done all you can do here today. I will turn this in for you, and you can go home."

It didn't seem right that this adventure at DHS should end so quickly. We were expecting to see someone to get some answers and establish a plan. But now, it was back to the waiting room at home and we still didn't know anything.

Linda and I went down to the ground floor and left the building. I wasn't sure if we accomplished anything or not.

"Wow, we were only here thirty minutes," Linda said.

"We can be thankful that God was with us, but three weeks? Do you think the hospital will be okay with that?"

"Well we weren't here all day like we thought we would be, and we were going to the hospital later this week anyway. I feel okay, so let's go on over there now and talk to them."

"But we don't know what to tell them," I said.

"We will tell them what DHS told us," she said.

So we headed for Hillcrest Hospital where the surgery would take place. We didn't know if they would let us in without insurance or some other kind of plan. Everywhere we went for medical reasons, the first question we were asked was always, "Who is your insurance carrier?" Well, we did sort of have a plan. The only problem with our Medicaid plan was, it was three weeks away, and we didn't know what the outcome would be. The Cancer Care Center made it sound like this would be easy, and we thought we could do it all in one day. To us, it seemed that Satan was still trying to cause problems. I thought of 1 John 4:4, "Greater is He that is in you than the one who is in the world."

We arrived at Hillcrest, and I stopped at the patient drop-off area. We gave thanks to God that we lived in a time with great medical knowledge and not a hundred years ago. We asked God for His help while we were there as He had helped us at DHS.

Linda got out of the car and made it to the chairs just inside the doors. I parked the car and found a wheel chair to make the trip easier for her. We found the admitting office and told them our doctor sent us to make arrangements for the April first surgery. They led us straight to the finance department for our first stop. We sat in the hallway among six small offices.

I have no idea about the cost, I thought. *Is it twenty thousand or one hundred twenty thousand? We will have ten or twelve medical facilities wanting payments costing more than a car. I don't care about the cost,* I kept telling myself. *I want my wife well. If we need more money, I know God will provide it—somehow.*

Satan can play some tricks on us when it comes to money. We never think we have enough. We don't like to give it up. Some places (like hospitals) won't talk to you if you don't have any. Satan may have some tricks, but I know it is not in God's plan for any to be sick. Jesus healed all who came to Him. Jesus came to do God's will, not His own (John 6:38). We would just have to go in this office knowing God was in charge.

A lady came out of one of the offices and called us in. The name plaque on the desk said Kathy.

Kathy walked behind her desk. "How can I help you?" she asked.

We told her of the ovarian cancer and the surgery scheduled for April first by Dr. Kevin.

"Who is your insurance carrier?"

"We have no insurance," I quietly told her.

This was where the trouble usually started, so we laid out our plan to somehow pay later and our desperate need for the operation. We told her we were working with Social Security, and we only found out about all of this three days ago.

With every question she asked, I felt like we were going the wrong way.

Then she asked, "Have you been to the Department of Human Services for some help?"

Linda and I looked at each other and said, "We just came from there. We filled out papers, but they said it would be about three weeks before we hear from them, and that's after April first."

Kathy said, "That's fine. I will put you down as Medicaid pending," then she leaned back in her chair as if we were done.

"Does this mean I can have my operation?" Linda asked.

"Oh yes. We would never tell you that we can't help you," Kathy said.

"I was afraid you wouldn't operate on me without insurance."

Linda cried even harder than she had on the Friday when we found out she had cancer. Were these tears of joy and relief? Linda felt like she had no chance of getting proper care. Now she suddenly had great hope, and her faith was lifted. She knew she now had a chance. I think her energy level went up about 40 percent.

"I get to have my operation!" She said as she looked at me through tear-filled eyes.

Her joy was so overwhelming that I joined in with some of my own tears. I never imagined Linda was so worried about not getting medical help. In my mind I knew I would do anything possible even if I had to make payments the rest of my life. We both had a burden lifted off our hearts when we knew the operation would take place. We were working through a frightening disease, and God was helping us knock down our fears one at a time and we were ecstatic. Even Kathy appeared thrilled with Linda's joy.

We finished a little more paperwork after Linda and I calmed down. We still didn't have all the answers, but a great burden had been lifted off of the two of us. We told Kathy thank you, and we returned to our car and celebrated a little more.

"Did you see what happened in there?" I asked.

"God is leading us to all the right people."

"We have the best doctor we can get, and everything else falling into place."

"God is giving us His best."

The Bible tells us to give thanks for everything to God our Father in the name of our Lord Jesus Christ (Eph. 5:20). As we sat in the car, we paused for a moment just to say, "Thank you, Jesus."

We thought this would be a long, hard day, but it had only taken thirty minutes at the Department of Human Services and twenty minutes at Hillcrest. Linda felt better that day than she had in over a month. A great burden of worry, fear, and doubt had been removed from her, and a lot of my own had also been removed. We were still uncertain about a lot of things, but it looked a lot better that day than it did the day before.

We were close to Leslie's house, so we went over there to tell her about the events of the day. What a difference this day was compared to Friday when we learned about the cancer. And good news is always wonderful to share with the loved ones closest to you.

We returned home after our short visit with Leslie. We had no definite answers on anything yet, but we were simply putting our trust in God. He was with us that day without a doubt. We still had a little over a week before the surgery and a lot of places on our list from the Cancer Care Center to contact. There were places that might help with the drugs and a place to call that would provide a wig for when Linda's hair started falling out.

Linda made some phone calls the next few days. It was getting harder to do because she was becoming weaker each day. I couldn't help too much because they all wanted to talk to her. Social Security was the most important at this time. They tried to set up a meeting for April 6. Linda told them she would most likely still be in the hospital at that time and didn't know when she could come in. They sat up a phone interview for two in the afternoon about three weeks after the surgery.

Again we received a blessing. The interview with Social Security would be done on the phone, not in their office. I had a hard time believing that was possible, but we were seeing God at work in many ways.

April first, the day of surgery, was a day we were looking forward to. We were like a kid thinking his birthday would never arrive. We were on a countdown of days to get this garbage from Satan out of my wife.

"Just three more days," I said to Linda as we woke up Sunday morning.

"I can't wait!"

"Are you nervous?"

"A little bit."

"I would be. Do you want to go to church today?"

"I think so."

"If you get tired, I'll bring you home," I said. "What do you want for breakfast?"

I'm not a really good cook because I had never needed to be, but I was pretty good at breakfast. For a while, I would have to do all the cooking, cleaning, and shopping. I didn't mind the shopping too much or even the cooking, but I didn't care for the cleaning at all.

I fixed breakfast, and we went to the early church service. One of our friends at church said they would like to bring dinner to our house that night if that was okay.

"Okay! That is great!" I said with a bit of enthusiasm. "I won't have to cook."

We always invited the people offering food to join us for that meal. The fellowship was greater than the food. Our friends came over and shared a meal with us, taking care of everything. Dinner was placed in the oven to keep it warm until we were ready. We told them our story of the last few days: finding out about cancer, our trip to DHS and the hospital, and some of our fears.

When we started our meal, our conversation turned to the memories of our past— the ski trips we had made to Colorado, summer cookouts that had gone wrong, and our wonderful church family that brought us together so many years ago.

Our friends took care of clean up and put everything away. Linda and I were not allowed to help. It was wonderful to sit down with friends and talk about normal things instead of our troubles. It helped us to forget the circumstances we were facing for a few hours.

The night came to an end, our friends prayed for us and as they prayed, I realized why God did not heal

Linda in the first few days like we had hoped. If God had healed her, no one would really know but me, Linda, and God. We would tell a few, but many would not have seen anything miraculous. It would be soon forgotten. The road we were taking would allow the many people from our church and other churches that were helping to be witnesses to a healing in progress. Other believers would witness the love of Christ through us. They would see teamwork in the church. Our faith and the faith of our family and friends would be on display before those walking in doubt and unbelief. It was not just the healing that would glorify God, but the blessings of all the other things that would take place with speed and perfect timing. Years from now, some would be able to remember when Linda was healed from cancer. Linda and I would be a reflection of God's work for others to see.

We did not receive any definite answers on our finances that week, but we knew God was leading us. We knew surgery would take place. We knew God had our tomorrows figured out, and He would be there when we arrived. So we gave ourselves to Him, knowing He would somehow provide all our needs.

> Look at the birds of the air; they do not sow or reap or store away in barns, and yet your heavenly Father feeds them. Are you not much more valuable than they?
>
> Matt. 6:26

THE DAY OF SURGERY

It was the last day of March. March is the month of Linda's birthday. It was in March that she broke both her legs in a car accident many years ago. It was in March that she had her appendix taken out in the middle of the night. This year, it was the month that we learned of the cancer attacking her body.

"I think the third time is the charm," I said to Linda.

"What do you mean?"

"Well, you broke your legs in March, had your appendix removed in March, and now will have this surgery. If we skip March, you'll never get any older."

"Then I would never have a birthday. My kids would get older than me," she said.

"Yeah, I would hate to outlive my kids. Are you ready for tomorrow? Its April Fool's Day you know."

"I've been praying about it, but now I'm getting a little nervous," she said.

"So am I, but this is the way God chose to heal you. Look how many people have been affected by this already. I know we are going to be okay."

"I know, but I'm still a little scared."

"Yeah, I am too. God tells us not to worry. Why do you think we do it?"

"I don't know. Maybe we just want His answer right away."

"Or we wonder if He is going to answer," I said.

"Look at all God has done for us in the past. He has answered more than we asked."

"I know my past pretty well; He has pulled me out of a lot of fires."

"It is time to let Him pull us out of this fire."

She is right, I thought. I would still worry and I would still trust in His answer to come. I knew God would take care of us; I just didn't know how.

"I will trust Him with my childlike faith," I said. We spent the day with just the two of us except for a couple of phone calls. Some of the calls we did not answer because we did not want to. We talked, prayed, and read our Bibles. Linda was still attached to the couch with no desire to get up, so I fixed the meals and did what little work needed to be done that day. We retired to bed at about 10:30 p.m.

We had a good night's sleep before the day of surgery. We packed the car with a few things we prepared the day before. I could always go home if we needed anything else because we only lived fifteen minutes away. Linda was not allowed to eat, so we skipped breakfast and left for the hospital.

We were about to enter the admitting office when we found two of our good friends already there. We told everyone we had to be there at ten in the morning to check in, and the surgery would be around noon.

It was so wonderful to have brothers and sisters in Christ to be with us no matter what the circumstances.

These two friends sat with us through every bit of that day. And that day turned out to be much longer than we had hoped.

We went into the admitting office. Linda got tagged and banded and transported to the pre-op room. We all followed along laughing and joking, doing our best to make this feel like a regular day. She was placed on the bed they would use later to move her to surgery.

Before long, more friends and relatives showed up. It didn't take long before the crowd outgrew the little room we were in. We had to expand to a waiting room outside of the pre-op room. We each took turns for the next three hours so everyone could visit with Linda. No one talked about the surgery much. It was just a simple hysterectomy; they did this all the time. We all thought we would call it a day no later than four that afternoon.

The nurse gave Linda a shot at about one o'clock to make her relax. We gathered and had prayer for her, the doctors, and all others involved in this event.

Dr. Kevin came in about 1:15 p.m. to talk to Linda and me.

Linda reached for the doctor's hand and spoke to him, "I have prayed for you and your work on me. I want you to know as you work that I want to live. I want to see my grandkids."

Somehow I knew those words would stay with him the rest of the day.

They moved Linda to the surgery room about 1:30 p.m. Our group of visitors moved to the surgical waiting room. This was a big room with short walls to separate multiple families. We filled half of it.

The room had a volunteer worker that handled the incoming phone calls where reports were made to the family members. She kept track of who we were and where we were sitting. I was told a nurse would call about once an hour with a progress report on the surgery.

Our group gathered in a huddle and the minister of our church led us in a prayer. We took our seats and exchanged a few jokes and stories from our past. We got into our snacks and acted as if we did this all the time. I knew all those around me were filled with Jesus Christ, and I believed we were all there to build each other up. I would have hated going through this alone as some people do.

I was surrounded by friends who kept me from thinking ugly thoughts, but Linda was alone. I wanted that phone call. I wasn't really worried that first hour, but I kept my eyes and ears on the phone across the room. My biggest concern was I didn't want Linda to be alone. I would have stayed with her until the last minute if I could have.

The first phone call I received was at three o'clock. I was informed that other delays had taken place, and Linda was just beginning her surgery. I hoped she was on a sleeping pill or something so she wouldn't be lying there by herself all that time.

After talking to the nurse on the phone, I told our group, "They are starting the operation now. Not bad for a hospital, only three hours late."

I didn't really care what time it was, but I had to tell everyone something.

A few people had to leave and go back to work. Some new visitors were arriving. They asked if I was hungry and volunteered to go get something for me to eat.

"No," I said. "I might get something after the next report."

That day eating didn't seem so necessary. Plenty of people were bringing in snacks all day. I didn't really care for anything, but I did dig around in the snack bag for some dark chocolate a couple of times.

It seemed like a long time until the next phone call came in. Every time the phone would ring, everyone in the room would watch the volunteer worker in anticipation for a report about their loved ones. It was good for me to have so many friends around to keep me from thinking the worst thoughts or worrying about what was going on in the other room.

Our next phone report came in one hour like they said. It was a simple report and good to hear. I reported to the others, "Linda is doing fine, and the surgery is coming along well."

The next call came at about 5:45 p.m. I wanted to tell the nurse it had been over an hour and a half since the last call, but I thought it was wonderful that they would call us at all. The longer time between calls caused more concern, but this report was about the same.

"Linda is doing well, we have not had to give her any blood, and we will call again in about an hour," the voice said on the phone.

The calls were really nice. If we'd had to sit there until the surgery was over without any reports, I would have been going nuts by then.

I reported back to our group, "They said everything is fine and would call again in about an hour. If this is a three hour operation, the next call may be the last one."

I truly hoped the next call would be the last; I was ready for this to be over, and I wanted to see my wife. I looked around the room at all the people. Our group was always quiet when I came back from the phone. They were curious about the report. I noticed the same silence from the entire room each time the phone rang. *What power that phone has*, I thought. No matter where you are, if a phone rings, everyone looks or checks their cell phone. I remember the days when there was never a report until the surgery was over.

We had been in the surgical waiting room all afternoon. We had seen people from other families sit and cry all day. Some of them had no one to sit and stay with them. They were all alone. We reached out to some of those that would let us. We offered them some of our snacks. I asked some of them if they knew Jesus or needed prayer. We said prayers for those who would let us through the day, but most were happy just to have someone else care.

One man that heard us praying asked if we would pray for his needs also. It felt good to have someone see a reflection of Christ in my life. I thought about facing our problems that day without Jesus, and I would not want to try.

A lot of people face the problems that life brings, and they do it without Jesus. They always seem confused and worried. They don't have that safety net that Christians have. Yes, I was a little worried, and I knew my wife's life was at stake, but I also knew the outcome would be perfect and wonderful because we belong to Jesus. I knew without a doubt, we had a place in heaven (John 14:3), although we were not trying to go that day.

It had been a long day. At six o' clock, the volunteer worker made an announcement that her day was over, and she would be going home. Our own little group of prayer warriors was thinning, and except for about four other people in the waiting room, we were all that was left. Surgery for most had ended, and all future incoming phone calls would be for us.

I hadn't eaten all day except for a few bites of dark chocolate, so I went with my friend, Cheryl, to the hospital cafeteria. Other friends would listen for the call we needed from the phone hanging on the wall. I made sure someone had my cell phone number in case they needed to reach me, and I left with Cheryl for a quick bite to eat.

We had a few more visitors stop by on their way home from work expecting to find Linda in a recovery room.

"She is still in surgery," I would tell them. "Thanks for stopping by."

There was not a lot to do in a waiting room, and we had been waiting a very long time. I received the next report at 7:30 p.m. They said there was a little more work to do, and they did have to give her one unit of blood.

The next hour passed very slowly. We watched the last person in the waiting room leave who was not part of our group. We were fifteen minutes into the second hour, still waiting and still no calls. I guess I was a little more concerned because they had given Linda some blood. Nine o'clock came and went and still no calls. We had waited an hour and a half earlier that day, but now she had been in there so long.

At 9:15 p.m. I was wondering if I could call someone, but we had no one to ask. All we could do was wait. Our group was talking less, and all of us were filled with our own thoughts and concerns. *Do they call the surgical waiting room this late? Do they remember we are out here?*

I checked the phone to see if it was still working. It had a tone, and I quickly hung up in case they might call. I sat there staring at the phone like my own will could cause it to ring. *Please ring and say they are finished and Linda is fine.*

Then the phone rang, and I about jumped out of my skin. I didn't give it time to finish the first ring before I answered, "How is Linda?"

The nurse calling us said, "Linda is doing well and is in the recovery room. The doctor will be out to see you shortly."

I hung up the phone and looked at our group of about eight people. I could feel God's presence and knew He had been with us all day. I knew He was also with Linda and her doctors.

"Linda is doing well!" I reported to our crowd. "And she is in the recovery room. The doctor will be here soon to give us a report."

I could see relief on their faces, and I could see their smiles returning. We gave thanks to our Lord and began a new time of waiting. I wondered how she was doing. *Is she awake? Is she in any pain? How many hours a week does that doctor work? Has this been a long day for him?* He had been standing over my wife all day working on her insides. This three-hour operation had turned into almost seven hours. I was looking forward to his report but more so to seeing my wife.

Dr. Kevin came out to the waiting room a little after ten o'clock. He looked tired and I felt sorry for him. I knew this man had been there since ten o'clock this morning because he had another operation before my wife.

"Thanks for coming to see us, Doctor," I said as I pointed to our assembly. "This is my family. How is Linda doing?"

Everyone stood and gathered around the doctor in anticipation of a good account.

"She is in recovery and doing well. We did have to give her two units of blood this last hour," Dr. Kevin said. "We found the tumor bigger than we had expected. That is why the surgery took a little longer than usual. The tumor was trying to spread to other organs, but I took out ninety five percent of it. I removed her ovaries and uterus, which contained most of the cancer. The tumor had something like little fingers that were reaching out and touching some of the other organs. If

Linda were an older person, I would have closed at that time, but she is young and strong, so we kept working."

I thought this was where God held the words she spoke to him before surgery in his brain. I looked at my daughter Leslie and noticed her crying, so I immediately went to her side and gave her a hug. I joined her with tears of my own as we continued to listen.

The doctor went on to say, "I had to scrape the walls of some of the other organs to remove these fingers. The bladder is like a ball with a layer of skin on the inside and on the outside. I had to remove the skin on the outside. This skin will come back much like the skin on your arm if it is cut away. She will be hurting for a few days, so she is being given morphine to help with the pain. She will be staying in the hospital for about fourteen days."

Dr. Kevin gave a very lengthy report. I knew I did not get all of it. I knew I would see him every day for a while, and I still had a few questions.

"When can I see her?" I asked.

"You can go back to see her now, but no more than two at a time," he said. "She is still under the drugs and will not be able to talk. She has some tubes in her so don't be shocked when you see her. She is okay."

"What about the five percent you did not get out?" I asked.

Dr. Kevin said, "That will be taken care of with chemo which gets all the microscopic pieces we can't see with our eyes. We will talk about that in a few days."

Then he looked at me and said, "After you see her, go home and get some rest. You are going to need it. She will not know if you stayed here or not anyway."

I said, "I guess so," and we thanked him.

He said, "A nurse will be here shortly to take you to the recovery room," and he left.

I looked for my daughter. She was sitting down and was still crying. I sat beside her.

"I could have lost my mom tonight," she said.

"But you didn't," I said through my own tears.

"I didn't even know she had cancer," Leslie said.

It was at this moment I realized how much Linda and I had been in denial about the cancer. When we talked to others, we had been referring to it as the mass that was attached to Linda's uterus. We had not even used the word cancer in front of our kids.

"I'm sorry. I guess we were afraid to say the word. I want you to go with me to see her," I said.

Leslie and her mother are very close. I knew it would be hard for her to go see her mother at all, and I didn't want her to go alone. I was trying to be strong, but I didn't want to go alone either. It was good that we had each other.

Leslie was about four months pregnant with her second child and our fourth grandchild. This is the grandchild Linda was referring to when she said she wanted to hold her grandbaby. This one was no different than the other three, except that she hadn't held this one yet. The nurse came quickly, and Leslie and I followed her to the recovery room.

It took a few seconds to recognize that this was my wife. She had tubes and wires attached to her, and she was covered with sheets and pillows making her hard to see. As we got closer, she looked at us through eyes that could not stay open. She knew we were there and raised her hand. I took it into both of mine.

"You made it," I whispered to her. The doctor said she wouldn't know we were there. I was surprised by her actions.

She opened her mouth to speak, but I could hear nothing. I leaned over, placing my ear close to her mouth.

I could barely hear her, and she said, "Mice." At least, that's what I thought she said.

The nurse was watching and showed me a cup of ice with a spoon setting on the table.

"She wants some ice," the nurse said. "Give it to her now because she can't have any after we move her to her room."

I placed some of the crushed ice on her lips. I could tell it felt good to her. Leslie and I took turns doing this each time she would touch her lips with her finger. She did not try to talk anymore that night.

Another nurse came in and told us, "We will be moving Linda to her room in a few minutes. Please return to the waiting room, and we will come get you as soon as we move her."

Leslie and I headed back to the waiting room.

"Have you talked to your sister?" I asked her on the way.

Wendy had been in several times that day, but was at home for now waiting on a call.

"No. I don't think I can right now," she said.

I told her I would call, and Leslie returned to our group. I walked across the room out on a balcony where I could talk without being distracted. *I will be strong when I talk to her*, I told myself as I dialed the number on my cell phone.

"Hello," Wendy said.

"It's me," I said. "Your mom is out of surgery, and she looks fine." I felt like that wasn't quite true, but I didn't want to upset Wendy.

I was doing my best to relay the information the way a father should, but then I glanced back to the waiting room where I saw Leslie sitting in the chair in tears again. You just can't see your kids hurting like that. It does something to you. I broke down again too.

Wendy could tell over the phone I was struggling. I could barely talk. She is my strong daughter in times like this.

"Mom will be okay," she said, trying to comfort me.

"I know."

I could barely talk, but her calmness made me feel better. I could no longer look at Leslie either while I was on the phone. I turned my back to her and regained my composure the best I could and finished our conversation.

"Call me if I can do anything," my daughter said.

"I will."

I hung up the phone and thanked Jesus for both of my girls. They are so different from each other and yet somewhat alike. I stood there on the balcony a few more minutes waiting for my strength to come back, and then I returned to our much smaller group.

I told them, "They are about to move Linda to her room. You can stay if you want, but Linda really needs to rest. She can't talk, and she doesn't know you are here, but she is doing fine. I don't know if I will stay the night or not, but I will stay and see her to her room. You might as well go home and get some rest."

Everyone, including Leslie, went home except two people. It was the same two friends who were waiting for us to arrive at the hospital that morning. The three of us sat down to talk some more as we waited for Linda to be moved.

We waited for about twenty more minutes, and I told Cheryl, "You have been here longer today than I have. Why don't you go home and come up in the morning."

She gave me a hug and went home.

Another ten minutes passed, and I decided I had waited long enough. I made up my mind, I was going to go back there and stand beside my wife until they moved her to her room. I would not spend one more minute in this waiting room away from my wife.

I told my last remaining friend, "I have to go back in there. I can't wait any longer."

"I understand," he said.

We exchanged our last words for the night, he said a prayer for us, and he also went home. I was now alone in the waiting room.

We had many people come by that day. Some for an hour or two, some for eight or ten hours, but it was a very special friend who will stay for the whole trip no matter what. Fourteen hours they stayed. My friends went the extra mile for sure. They stayed with me the same as Jesus stays with us (Heb. 13:5).

I opened the door to go to the last place I had seen my wife and started walking down the hall. The surgery Linda needed was finally over, but the night was just getting started.

THE HOSPITAL STAY

I went back to the recovery room where Linda was waiting to be moved. I decided I would stay with her and give her ice as long as she wanted. It was half past midnight before Linda was rolled toward her hospital room. I walked next to her all the way, thinking I would go home and get some sleep after we got her settled in.

She was moved to a full-size bed by four attendants. All the tubes and hoses and wires were moved with her. They plugged her into a machine to monitor her blood pressure, heart rate, and other vital functions. Two of the attendants left and the two nurses for that floor stayed on duty for the rest of the night checking Linda every fifteen minutes. They worked from seven to seven so their day (or night) was only half over.

One nurse finished taking Linda's blood pressure, drew some blood, and left the room. The other nurse was fighting with the suction hose trying to get it to work. She sounded like she was having a hard time catching her breath. I thought she must be a smoker. How can you work in a hospital and be a smoker? Her name tag said Brenda.

I asked her, "Why is that suction hose in her nose?"

Brenda said, huffing and puffing, "It is to keep everything out of her stomach. The last thing you want right now is for her to be nauseous."

Brenda made a final connection to the hose and said, "That should do it."

I looked at it and said, "No, I don't think it is working."

She looked at it and said, "No, it's fine."

"I'm no doctor," I said, "but I have been an engineer all my life. This fluid is not moving in the hose, and I hear air coming in on that wall connection."

She looked at the bottle on the wall and said, "I think we're missing a piece up here. I'll get one from one of the other rooms," and she left to search for the missing piece.

Linda was holding my hand pretty tightly, I thought, for someone that was supposed to be half asleep and on morphine. She was also tapping her lips again with her index finger.

I whispered to her, "They said you couldn't have any more ice. I'll ask them again in a minute."

Brenda returned with a few plastic parts in her hand and some more tubing. She changed a few parts one way, and then another.

"That should do it," she said.

I heard those same words a minute ago. I looked at the hose.

"It's still not working," I said.

"This doctor does things a little different from the other doctors. This is how he likes it hooked up. I'll go check his orders again," she said as she left the room.

I don't know about doctor orders, but I knew this wasn't working and I wasn't leaving until it was.

Brenda came back in a few minutes and said, "This doctor's orders are very hard to read. I was supposed to hook this up as an intermittent suction. I'll have this fixed in a minute."

"Okay," I said. "Can my wife have some ice?"

"I don't know. I will check her file when I return to the desk," she said as she continued wrestling with the hose.

After a bit, Brenda said, "Now it is set up like the doctor wants it."

I looked. "It is still not working! Is that what the doctor ordered?" I said with a little sarcasm.

"Let me check that doctor's orders again," she said and hurried out of the room.

My thoughts at that time would not have sounded very Christian, so I kept my mouth shut. *I could fix it myself,* I thought. *I'm a pretty good engineer, but I might cause it to work better than it was intended.* I waited for repairs, but I didn't wait patiently.

Every once in a while we all find someone who is *not* the best at their job. It is a blessing for us that Brenda was the only one so far. Everyone else we encountered on this journey had been the best we could find. I believe that too was a blessing God had surrounded us with in our time of need. However, I was losing my control.

Brenda came back and said, "I read his orders wrong. Dr. Kevin wants a continuous suction."

This was where I lost any control and yelled at her, "I don't care what kind of suction he wants. Get someone in here that can make this thing work. I don't want my wife throwing up because you can't figure out how to make this thing work!"

To be honest, that sounded a lot better than what I was thinking. It takes a lot to make me mad unless it is about my wife or my kids, but I got the point across, and I was more than glad I didn't go home like the doctor had told me to do. Much of his work could have come undone if this hose did not function properly.

It wasn't long before someone from the recovery room came back to fix the suction machine. None of the machine was properly set up and a few parts were still missing. They told me that this floor seldom had any use for this type of equipment so they were not familiar with it.

"If you don't know the equipment, you shouldn't be acting like you do and saying everything is fine," I said.

I was still a little upset, but I could see some suction starting to work.

"Everything is working as it should be now," the man said. "Let us know if you need anything else."

I thanked him and there was no more trouble with the suction hose. I did have a talk with the hospital floor supervisor the next morning.

The other nurse came in to check blood pressure again. I was glad it wasn't Brenda.

I asked this nurse if Linda could have some ice. Her mouth was so dry.

She said, "No, but I'm not sure why. Everything is being pumped out of her stomach anyway."

The nurse gave us a bag of sticks that had a small sponge on the end.

"You can dip this in water and use it to keep her lips wet," she said.

I was told earlier that Linda would not know if I was there or not. I also thought she would sleep. She didn't sleep, and she didn't want me to go home, which she made clear. She didn't talk either, but she knew how to keep that wet sponge attached to her lips. I knew how the disciples felt in Mark 14:37. I was going to be keeping watch with Linda all night, and there would be no sleep for me. Someone was checking something every fifteen minutes for the rest of the night. I had a futon next to Linda's bed, but I only sat on it a few times.

When seven in the morning came around, the shift change took place, and we received a new crew of nurses. We didn't see Brenda again while we were there. Linda finally started to fall asleep. The new nurse who came in told me they would now be checking on her once every hour.

Linda is greatly loved at our church and outside of our church. I did not want anyone to see her until we were both ready. I went to the main desk on this floor and put a password in the system, which is usually done for patients who have overdosed on drugs so that their friends can't bring in more drugs. I did it to prevent visitors. The hospital would inform anyone asking for Linda that they have no one with that name. Under the password protection rule, you must give the patient's name and the password to get the room number. They do not ask you if you know the password.

I called my daughters and my close friends who stayed the fourteen hours with us and gave them the password and the room number. Even if you had the room number, you still needed the password. The women's hospital wing that Linda was in had locked doors on each floor. Security had to open the door, and in Linda's case, you also needed the password.

I hoped this would not make anyone at our church mad, but I also thought if they really loved Linda, then they would understand. Besides, I would take all the heat, and I was giving reports to the church. I did tell our church I had placed a password on Linda and told them not to come for a visit at that time because the hospital wouldn't let them in. I also said I would remove the password as soon as I could.

After breakfast I stopped at the main desk near the entrance to the hospital on my way back to Linda's room. I asked them for the room number.

The girl looked Linda's name up on the computer and told me, "We have no one with that name here."

"Good," I said. "The password is working. Thank you."

I waved goodbye to her and went on my way back to the room hoping I would not have any trouble getting back through the security doors on that floor. They opened the doors as soon as they saw me and let me in.

Dr. Kevin came in around nine that morning. He checked, probed, and listened as doctors do. He told us everything looked good and reminded us that it would be about two weeks before she could go home.

The doctor said, "I want Linda up and walking around today."

I looked at him like he must be crazy.

"She can walk to this chair and sit up for a few hours," he said as he pointed next to the bed.

I told him, "We will try."

"Have you been here all night?" he asked.

I must have looked like I hadn't had any sleep, or maybe he knew I had on the same clothes.

"Yes," I said and told him about Brenda.

He said he would talk to the floor supervisor about it as he left the room. I didn't tell him I had already done that, but I also thought it would be better coming from him.

By about one o'clock in the afternoon, Linda was able to work the sponge stick by herself if I propped up the Styrofoam cup in the right place. She had learned to soak the sponge completely and draw out every drop of water. She wasn't allowed to have a drink, but found a way to drain that cup about every twenty minutes. She was also over-working the morphine button they gave her to inject herself, and she was beginning to whisper a little louder.

She told me, "Thank you for staying last night. I needed you here."

That's not what her doctor told me last night, I thought.

"You knew I was here?" I said.

"Yes. I heard you fighting with the nurse. Thank you."

"It wasn't much of a fight," I said. "It was simply going to be fixed one way or the other. I'm going to go home and get cleaned up, and then we will try to get you into that chair."

"Okay."

She hit the morphine button one more time and closed her eyes to sleep. I refilled her Styrofoam cup, put in a fresh sponge stick, and left to go home.

Calls were starting to come in on my cell phone asking if I had moved Linda. Everyone was being told she was not in this hospital. Over the next few hours as I cleaned up, I had to explain many times I was restricting visitors for now. I would remove the password in a few days when Linda was able to have visitors.

As I passed through our bedroom to finish getting dressed, I paused at the edge of our bed. *That sure looks good,* I thought. It had been a long time since I'd gone this long with no sleep. I was looking forward to some time in that bed tonight, but right then, I had to get back to the hospital.

With the help of two nurses, we worked on moving Linda to the chair to sit up for a while. I removed the massage wraps from her legs. They were there to help prevent blood clots. The nurses were arranging all the tubes to the side of the bed with the chair. The nurses did most of the work because I was afraid to help. It was her first time out of bed, and it wasn't easy. With a lot of pain, (some of it mine) Linda was moved to the chair. I think she would have been happier to stay in the bed a few more days, but once she was in the chair for a few minutes and caught her breath, she was good for about two hours.

Two of our friends with the password came for a visit, and so did our daughters, of course. Leslie, my youngest daughter, gave us $140 that her Sunday school class had taken up for us. They wanted to help me with meals and gas while Linda was in the hospital. It was another surprise blessing from being in the family of God. My daughter goes to a different church than Linda and I, but we all are in God's family, and they wanted to help.

The rest of the day went without any problems except for moving from the chair back to the bed. It was about as painful as moving from the bed to the chair. Visiting hours ended on our first full day in the hospital, and I was trying to go home myself, but Linda did not want me to leave. She told me she was scared to stay alone. I think the morphine was having strange effects on her.

I stayed with her again that night. I had already gone about forty hours with no sleep, so I turned off all the lights I could and laid on the futon for some rest. The once-an-hour, nursing calls made sleep difficult. Sometimes they needed more light, sometimes they were noisy, but I was always awake and watching. We had a very good gathering of nurses for the rest of Linda's stay. Sometime during the night, one of the nurses covered me with a blanket I did not have when I laid down. I must have slept through one of the hourly calls.

The next morning, I watched Linda, and she slept until afternoon. *She plays a big part of fellowship in our church*, I thought. She was always there serving the people at many of the gatherings we have. She had been greatly missed these last two months, and there would be many more months to come that she would be missed. I realized how much she meant to other people, not just to the kids and me.

So why was she, or anyone, faced with a sickness or disease that disrupts the lives of so many people? Why was Satan trying to take her out with cancer? Why would he do that? He knew he couldn't have her. He knows she belongs to God.

I thought about the time in the Bible when Satan attacked Job. Like Linda, Job was a good person (Job 1:1). He was a powerful man that owned much, yet why would our perfect and loving God allow so much destruction to fall on someone?

I opened my Bible on my Blackberry and started reading Job in chapters one and two. Job was a righteous man. It appeared God was giving permission to Satan to attack Job. I had come to believe that if you truly love the Lord and trust in Him in all things, then He will give good and perfect gifts (James 1:17).

I knew my wife, and she did believe and live for the Lord. Then I read Job 3:25-26 and realized I did not know Job. I cannot see what another person is thinking, but Job said that what he had feared the most had happened to him. What he dreaded most had come true.

Job did fear the Lord, but he also had doubt that God would take care of him (James 1:6). I knew that

Linda had no doubt that God would take care of her. So I looked again at my sleeping wife, wondering, *Why is she being attacked?* I also knew God is patient and would give me the answers I was searching for in time.

The next few days were very hard. Linda hurt each time she tried to get up and walk. We would move the bed to many different positions and shapes trying to make her feel better. One day, as she sat in the chair near the bed, I took her place in the bed. It made no difference where it was adjusted to; it didn't feel good. There was a large void in the middle of the mattress. I tried stuffing it with pillows or blankets. I tried putting pillows under the mattress. It was a hindrance she was going to have to live with until we left. The nurse told us that the women's wing had the best beds in the hospital. If that was true, I really felt sorry for all the other people staying in this building.

We were getting ready for one of our walks. It wasn't easy. I had to take off her leg massage wraps, hang the Foley on the IV pole, disconnect the suction hose, wind up all other tubes, and get a nightgown on Linda. It was about as far as a football field to walk around the inner rooms of our floor. Linda always held on to her IV pole for balance as we walked. She walked very slowly, but was doing well.

I began taking very large and slow steps, entertaining myself at this slow pace. I had taken about two steps in a slow motion fashion when Linda stopped walking and closed her eyes.

"Stop that! It scares me," she said.

I laughed. "How can that scare you?"

"I have seen people walking slow in my dreams, and I don't like it."

I didn't do that anymore, but I realized she had been scared ever since that first night. It must have been the side effects of the morphine, and the side effects were affecting me too. It had been keeping me in the hospital every night.

On the fourth day, the vacuum hose going into Linda's stomach was removed. I found her sitting in her chair smiling when I returned from lunch. Not only was she much happier, but she could eat real food. I lifted the security password so that we could allow the grandchildren and all the visitors from our church to come in. It is amazing how much better things are without a tube in your nose and with a visit from your grandkids.

On the fifth day, Linda was going for a walk every hour or two. We took a walk to the other end of the hospital where we had not been before. We found the nursery, which had about thirty babies in it. Babies are always good for bringing out the best in Linda. She laughed and talked about memories of our own kids, but soon remembered her own situation.

"I want to go home," she said.

"I know you do, but I don't think I can take care of you yet."

"I am scared in here, and I have bad dreams."

"It's the morphine," I told her. "And I have been here with you every night."

"I know, and I'm glad you have been here. I don't know how I would do this without you."

We returned to the room, got Linda back in bed, and prayed for the morphine to be removed. It is amazing how God is always ahead of us in our wants and our needs. He takes care of those who seek Him (Matt. 7:7).

Dr. Kevin came in that afternoon and removed the morphine supply line and put her on a different pain medication. This was another blessing from God. Right after Linda and I had talked and prayed about this problem, it was removed. Not only was that problem fixed, but a few hours later, the nurse came in and removed the tube feeding into the back of her hand. The needle was still in, but she now had freedom from the IV pole.

We gave thanks again to Jesus Christ for so many blessings in one day.

Later, two of our friends came walking in with a plastic bucket about thirty gallons in size. The bucket was from our Sunday school class and was full of crackers, cookies, chips, sodas, and other great snacks. They told us it was for us and our visitors.

"Visitors!" I said. "Are you crazy? I'm going to eat all of this stuff."

Our friends know I have a weakness for dark chocolate, and there was a bag in there just for me. I laid the snacks out for others to have, but I kept the bag of dark chocolate in hiding.

It was a wonderful thing for us the day we joined God's family. We know and believe Jesus Christ is the Son of God (John 3:16) and Jesus Christ is the only way to heaven (John 10:7, John 14:6). Our friends were our family, and we all have the same Father.

Linda was doing so well, and on the seventh day, around five o'clock in the evening, Dr. Kevin came in and told Linda she could go home tonight if she wanted. I had not seen her look that happy since she received her most recent grandchild.

"Okay, Doc," I said, "but what about that catheter? Are you going to take it out?"

"No, she will need it a few more weeks until her bladder can heal," he said.

"I guess a few weeks won't be too bad. My father-in-law will have one for the rest of his life."

So okay, I was going to take Linda home with a catheter and a tube with a small ball still attached to the incision in her stomach. She couldn't cook or do most anything by herself. I wouldn't be able to leave the house. It had been seven days, not fourteen. Now the fear of what falls on me was becoming a reality, and it was a little frightening.

"Okay, I can do this. I did it when she had two broken legs," I said.

I had been watching all week so I knew how to drain the little incision ball thingy, and I could pull the plug on the Foley. As long as she doesn't have any problems, I knew I'd make it.

Dr. Kevin said, "I will schedule a nurse to come by your house three times a week."

That, I thought, *was a good plan*. Last time I took care of Linda with her broken legs, my mother-in-law and father-in-law moved into our house for about two months. They are very good people, and we needed their help, but we prefer a visit.

The doctor said he would start the release papers and would be back shortly. Then he left the room.

"Wow, we're going home," I said, hoping I didn't sound too nervous.

"I don't think I could sleep in this lumpy bed another week," Linda said. "You have no idea how much I want my own bed."

"I think maybe I do. That futon is not the best place to spend the night with the lights going off and on all night. It will be good for both of us to get some real sleep."

We started making plans and packing all her things. It was amazing how many things had been brought in for her—food, new clothes, flowers, and cards—and there were things the hospital provided for us to take home. I made two trips to the car and had one more load to take on our way out.

"You call the girls, and I will call the church to let them know we are moving out of here," I told her as I packed everything else I could find.

I, on the other hand, was still wondering how I would handle all this. *What am I to do if something goes wrong? I'm an engineer, not a medical assistant. I could fix a suction hose, but I couldn't fix Linda*. After an hour had passed, I realized I shouldn't be so worried, and we waited some more. I don't think we ever get use to waiting; we just tolerate it because we have to.

Another hour had passed and the doctor had still not returned.

"Do you think he forgot and went home?" Linda asked.

"I doubt it. He's a busy man. I'll go check the hall."

He was sitting behind a computer at the main desk filling out reports and entering data. I wondered if the man ever got to spend any time with his own family. I had seen him here early in the morning and late in the evening. He has an office that is open five days a week. I don't think I would want to be a doctor.

I went back to the room and said, "He is still here."

We waited and another hour passed. I was starting to receive calls on my cell phone from those who thought we would be at home. My patience isn't the best, but I started thinking, maybe Linda should wait until morning. It was getting late, and we were both tired.

Dr. Kevin came back about 9:30 p.m. He is a very good doctor, but he reminds me of one of my good friends. I think my friend does not understand a clock. He lives in his own world and doesn't know that time exists. If he says eight in the morning on Tuesday, he means sometime before three in the afternoon.

"I'm sorry I took so long. I had a patient in the next room with a small emergency. You can go home tonight if you want, but it might be better to wait until morning," he said.

We decided to wait, because it would take until midnight if we went tonight. More of the people we needed to help us check out would be there in the morning.

Linda was over the effects of the morphine, and she took pity on me and told me to go home for the night. We were both ready for bed, so I kissed her goodnight, grabbed another sack of stuff going to the car, and went home to get some sleep. Tomorrow, Linda would come home. It would be like a sheep without a shepherd because I did not know what to do. For us a new way of life would begin.

THE HOMECOMING

I arrived at the hospital around seven the next morning. I was rested now and felt a lot more confident in bringing Linda home. Dr. Kevin was expected around eight. I found Linda already sitting in her chair waiting on breakfast.

"Did you get there by yourself?" I asked.

"No, but I couldn't stay in that bed anymore," she said. "I can't wait to get home and sit on my couch and lie on my own bed."

"I'm ready to stay home for a while too," I said.

As we waited for the doctor, we talked about how we thought life would be the next few weeks. We really didn't know; we'd never had cancer in our house. We have seen others with cancer, but we don't know how life was in their house. We knew we would be better off than some because we have Christ in our lives. Each day would be brand new for us, and we would have to trust in God. We didn't know what to expect, and we were still looking for a way to pay for all this.

I said, "Well, we just have to put it in God's hands."

Dr. Kevin came in about 9:30 a.m. to give us final directions before setting us free. He started with directions for Linda.

"You are not allowed to pick up anything over four pounds, and you need to walk around a little bit each day," he told her. "Also, call my office and make an appointment for next week as soon as you get home."

The rest of the directions were not for Linda, but for me.

"You will take care of all the shopping, cleaning, cooking, and anything else Linda points to. Watch her finger because that is all I want her to pick up. If you have to go somewhere, have someone stay with her. I will send a nurse to your house three times a week to help with medical needs."

We both thanked him, and he left. All we needed now was the final check out papers so the nurse could wheel Linda down to the patient pickup area. We waited. At 11:30 a.m., we were thinking about lunch when the nurse came in with a wheel chair. I had taken most everything down to the car already, but the hospital was giving us more stuff. I figured it would somehow be on the bill, so we loaded it into a bag. We were in a hurry to get home and get out of the hospital seven days sooner than expected.

The nurse told me to go move my car to the pickup area, and she would bring Linda to me. I left in a hurry to get there ahead of them so they would not have to wait on me, and I waited another twenty minutes in the car before they came. When I saw them coming, I jumped out of the car, loaded a few more things from Linda's lap, and began helping her into the car. We got her in and then I saw that Foley thing lying on the ground. I wasn't sure what to do with it, but I knew it had to go with us, so I tossed it in the car. *They really should give directions with these things,* I thought.

I ran around the car and got in behind the wheel.

"Where do you want to go?" I said.

"How about home?"

"What! You don't want to go to the mall or the amusement park or something?" I asked in a teasing voice.

"No. Just home please," she said.

I started heading down the hospital drive. We did not get very far before I quickly learned not to bounce the car at the first speed bump. Linda had around forty staples holding her together. All of the organs that she kept were still moving around searching for a place to stay in the extra space provided. She was very tender.

This is not going to be an easy trip, I thought. The roads around here are full of chug holes, and we live in the country. I'm a speedy driver, and I get a little upset with other drivers that need a bumper sticker that says Drivers in Training. It looked like I would be the slow, irritating driver that day.

Right in front of us, there it was. I couldn't go around it. We were at the end of the drive, and there was another speed bump. I touched it with the front tires from a dead stop. I gently gave the car a little gas, but it wouldn't go. I gave a little more gas, and the car started to climb. *Why do they make them so big?* When the tires finally climbed to the top of the bump we shot off the other side like a bottle rocket. I'm not sure if the tires left the ground, but Linda's shrieking was only a little short of cracking the windshield.

A simple bump or chug hole I used to ignore made me feel as if I were punching Linda in the stomach as we crossed it. This trip usually takes fifteen minutes, but this time, it took thirty. Most of the trip was on the highway, and I could travel full speed there, but our quarter-mile-long gravel driveway might have been faster to walk. It was filled with plenty of low spots and bumps I never noticed until that day.

Linda held herself together with both hands as I drove that last quarter mile over the rough terrain. I parked the car as close as I could to the front porch steps, got Linda out of the car, walked her up the two stairs and got her into the house and on the couch. I worked with the pillows and blankets to make her as comfortable as I could.

"Here we are," I told her. "We're finally home, and you're all tucked into your couch. Now, since you didn't want to stop on the way home, what can I fix you for lunch?"

She had no restrictions on food, which was good because I am not the best cook. I could do breakfast and hamburgers on the grill, and that's about it. Linda knew it too.

"How about a cheeseburger?" she said, trying to make it easy on me.

"Cheeseburger it is."

This is easy, I thought, *but what about dinner and tomorrow and after that?* I could live on cheeseburgers, but Linda would get tired of them really quick. I couldn't afford to drive to town two or three times a day for something else. *I guess I will have to learn to cook.*

It can't be too hard to follow the directions on a box or in a cookbook. I can build almost anything including dinner.

We had our cheeseburgers, and then I spent the next five hours cleaning up the kitchen. Not from making cheeseburgers, but because no one had been home in a week, and the mess was much older than I care to admit. Not much of anything had been done around the house for at least a month. I washed dishes, did a little laundry, threw out some old food from the fridge, organized the pantry to my liking, mopped the kitchen floor, made a shopping list, and prayed for some strength and some help.

I was far from finished; it would take many days. But now it was time to try to make something for dinner. The rules of the kitchen seemed to be making a mess, clean it up, make another mess, and clean it up again.

Linda decided she wasn't hungry and just wanted some cheese and an apple. Wow! That was easy. I had a sandwich on some bread that was a few days past the "use by" date and was glad to have the night off after cleaning all day. I think she was having pity on me.

We watched a little television, and at about nine o'clock that evening, we were ready for bed. By then, I had already slept an hour or so in my chair anyway. I walked Linda to the bathroom and had my first attempt at draining the Foley. I knew I was going to be glad to get rid of this thing, but I'm sure Linda would be even more excited than me.

We took care of a few other things and after about thirty minutes, Linda was in bed. We have a big bed, but I was afraid to stay in it because I might bump her in the night. I am an active sleeper, so I decided for another week or so I would sleep in one of the other bedrooms, like I did when her legs were broken.

"Holler if you need me," I said and I left the room.

We started our first full day in our house at seven the next morning. We were learning a new routine. Each day started with draining the Foley and the drainage bulb in the incision. No training came with these devises. I guess I should have asked, but I did watch all of this for a week at the hospital.

Each day I learned some new task I would need to take care of for a while. That morning, I made French toast for breakfast. It's pretty easy: soak a slice of bread in an egg, fry it in a pan, and add a little butter and syrup. I brought it to Linda on a tray with a glass of milk and a small bowl of grapes. She cried like a baby. I still don't know why today. Maybe it didn't look good; maybe she was surprised I could cook. I like to think it was because it was so much better than hospital food or maybe that she was amazed at my great kitchen talents. Who knows?

After breakfast, I returned to what was now *my* kitchen and cleaned up the mess so I could be ready to do it again in a few hours. I went through the pantry and other cabinets throwing out everything that was out of date. With all the chemicals and preservatives in everything today, a cupcake can last longer than a pregnancy, but I still threw out a trash can full of stuff.

Some of it I found in the freezer and just didn't know what it was.

This was the way life was in our house for a few days. The vacuum wouldn't work until I put in a new bag. The clothes would always spark and stick together coming out of the dryer and no one ever told me what kind of soap to put in the dishwasher. If you think your spouse doesn't have much to do, try doing it yourself for a month or two.

After a few hours of housework, I sat down in my easy chair. Looking out our front storm door, I could see little finger prints from my granddaughter as high as she could reach. I thought how nice it would be to have her come and visit again.

"We have a new problem," I told Linda.

"What?"

"We need groceries."

"We should have plenty in there," she said.

"We do. But I don't have a clue how to fix any of it. I have to go get something that I can fix."

We made a list of a few things Linda wanted and tried to list some things I might be able to cook. I decided I would just have to figure it out in the store.

Linda called a friend to come and visit with her so I could go. Before we belonged to a church, we didn't have as many friends. If life ever gives you a time of difficulty like cancer does, you need two things—a lot of friends to help and Jesus Christ. We had many occasions when we needed a visitor while I took care of other business. It always did Linda a lot of good to see someone besides me all the time too.

Another wonderful thing about God's family is they want to help. Many people from our church and my daughter's church would bring an evening meal to our house. Most would call ahead and ask if they could bring something on a certain day. We always invited them to bring plenty and sit and eat with us. This was one of the highlights of our hard times while being confined to our house. It was so wonderful to spend an evening with our brothers and sisters in Christ. We got to know some of our guests for the first time with that meal, and I didn't have to cook. You don't have to have a crisis or be sick to meet with old friends and discover new friends in your house.

I returned home with our groceries, most of them were pop-in-the-oven-then-sit-and-wait meals. This is not the healthiest way to eat, but it was a way I could handle. I also made sure we had paper plates to cut back on clean-up time. After all, my trash can is bigger than my dishwasher and a lot less work.

Marsha, from the home nursing staff, had already arrived for her first visit. Marsha was a short, little, black woman full of talk. She was very heavy for her height, and I know it had to be from the many pie recipes she told us about. Her family used to have a pie store, and she knew how to make them all.

"I like pie!" I got those words in between hers as she named about thirty pies.

"I'll make you a caramel pecan," she said as she glanced at me and waved her hand. She did not stop talking as she continued taking blood pressure and applying medical devices to Linda.

I watched and listened as that was all I could do. Linda was able to talk to her, but to me it was as if both were talking at once. I guess it's a woman thing. I just sat back in my chair thinking, *I like caramel pecan pie.*

When Marsha finished with her medical duties and thirty more minutes of chatter, she got up to leave. Then she saw some pictures of our grandkids on the wall. She and Linda talked another fifteen minutes about grandkids. When they finished, I walked with her out to her car. She talked all the way and told us she would be back in two days. I didn't say a word. I couldn't. I just stood in the front yard and waved at her as she drove off.

I returned to the house, and Linda said "She was really nice. I like her."

"Well, what did she say?"

"Oh, we had a nice talk about our kids and grandkids…"

"No," I interrupted, "I mean about your health."

"Oh, I'm fine," she said. "I look forward to her coming back."

"Well, I guess she will be here three times a week. That's more pie than we can eat."

Linda laughed and said, "I don't think she will bring you a pie every trip."

It was good to see Linda in a happy mood again. This was something that hadn't happened often for a long time. She still wasn't moving around too much, but Marsha and other visitors helped Linda to feel better.

The first week had passed, and it was time for Linda to leave the house for her first appointment with Dr. Kevin. I was a little worried about this—not about the doctor, but about the trip. She still had all those staples, and she was still sore. It was about forty miles to his office. I remember the very slow trip home and a couple of monster speed bumps. Will it be a slow trip this time?

First thing we had to do was get Linda ready. She had been wearing pajamas for a week (not the same ones) and now we needed to change to real clothes. That was the easy part. Our first problem was changing that giant Foley bag to the smaller bag that straps on her leg. It couldn't be too hard; the nurses do it all the time. But I had not seen this done. I got out all the parts, laid them on the floor, and put my engineering mind to work.

This leg bag had never been used, so I strapped it too her leg and cut the elastic straps to length. So far, so good. The tubing appeared to just slide off the big bag and on to the leg bag. The tube came off okay, but it would not stay on the leg bag. It kept popping off because the plastic connector was a different size.

"Bob, you have to fix this. I'm not going to the doctor carrying this thing around with me," she said.

"Hang on a minute; you know I can fix anything. I'll go get my vice grips and some wire. I'll make it work."

I didn't of course, but after probing through all the plastic parts and different size tubing I found a combination that would work, but the tubes were all too long. I did not want to cut any original tubing because

I needed to return all of this to the same configuration it started in when we came back home. I finally got everything worked out without using my hammer or the power saw.

"We need to see about picking up a few spare parts for this thing when we get to the doctor's office," I said. "That way I won't have to make any. Try not to forget, okay."

"Trust me, I won't forget."

We finished getting ready, and I walked Linda out to the car. It was much easier getting around now than it was last week. She was still hurting from the surgery, but in a different way from last month when the cancer was eating her insides. We knew that the healing process was underway. If you cut your finger, it heals in a few days, but even that is an act of God. He made our self-repairing skin. Everything around us is clearly made by the hand of God. God said if you open your eyes and look, you have no excuse for not knowing Him and His works (Romans 1:20).

We started out of our gravel driveway, and I could tell it would be better than the drive home last week. I took the bumps slower than usual, and Linda kept her hands on her stomach as if she were holding herself together. I asked God for a safe trip and a good report as we left our drive (Heb. 13:6).

I got Linda out of the car and into the seats just inside the glass doors where she could wait for me to park the car. When I returned, she had moved to the seats near the waterfall. I remembered when we came in here for the first time nearly a month ago, I thought we might sit here and talk later when we had more time. We had a few minutes, so I sat down beside her.

"I wonder what God has planned for me?" she said.

"Well, you've got to take care of me."

"No. You can do that yourself."

"You have plenty to take care of at church. You've been doing that a long time," I said.

"What I have been doing is fine, but what is next after cancer?"

"Who knows," I said. "God planned a big job for the apostle Paul before he was even born," (Gal. 1:15-17) "and Jeremiah while he was still in the womb," (Jer. 1:5).

"Those were big jobs," she said.

"How big of a job do you want? I can make taking care of me a big job," I joked.

"I just don't know what is going to happen or what to do next."

"It's not time for you to worry about that," I said as I pulled out my Blackberry and opened it.

I found the Bible verses I wanted to read to her where the writer was talking to God, and I read these words;

> I praise you because I am fearfully and wonderfully made; your works are wonderful, I know that full well. My frame was not hidden from you when I was made in the secret place. When I was woven together in the depths of the earth, your eyes saw my unformed body. All the days ordained for me were written in your book

> before one of them came to be. How precious to me are your thoughts, O God! How vast is the sum of them!
>
> Psalms 139:14-17

"Before you were born," I added, "God had a plan for you. It wasn't cancer. And when we get through this and the time is right, He will show you some more of His plans for you. He has a predetermined plan for every one of us, but some will not seek God's plan. His plan for you now might be to show others how to handle a crisis."

I put my phone away and jokingly said, "But I still think you need to take care of me. Let's go see Dr. Kevin."

When the doctor came in, he sat on the roll-around stool in front of our chairs to talk to us. After the small talk, "How do you feel?" and "You look good," he told us what to expect next.

"I am going to start you on chemo in May at the hospital. Get with my schedulers before you leave. They will have all the dates and times you need. Everything will be scheduled for one month in advance."

"How long will this last," Linda asked.

"There will be at least six treatments with three weeks between each one and we will see if more are needed after that. Have you had the chemo class that is given every week near the hospital?" he asked.

"No."

"My schedulers will give you that information too. You should bring all your family that is interested in taking the class with you. All your questions should be answered there. One thing you should know is that chemo is not the same as it was twenty years ago. It is now targeted towards your type of cancer. There are hundreds of different cancers, and the chemo best suited for you will be the one we will use. First, I want you to call the hospital. I have made an appointment for you next week to get a port put in."

"What is a port?" I asked.

"It is a small funnel that goes just under the skin on your chest," as he pointed to himself, "with a tube that comes across and is attached to the blood vessel coming out of your heart. This will be used for all future treatments instead of the IV needle in your arm. We can use this to draw blood and give chemo. It is faster and much easier for you. We could do all this through your arm, but the vessels in your arms are small and could be damaged from all the chemo."

"How long can this funnel stay in me?" Linda asked.

"It may be in there for years. It doesn't matter. It will be removed when we are sure we are done."

"I have two screws in my knee from a broken leg seventeen years ago," Linda said.

A nurse knocked on the door and entered with a stainless steel table on wheels.

"We may or may not keep the port that long," he said. "But right now, let's get you up on the table and take a look at those staples."

The nurse that came in and the doctor went to work. Dr. Kevin would pull a staple or two with a tool that looked like a pair of pliers. The metal staple would do a back bend and slip right out. I wondered how they were put in. He then put on strips of tape about a half inch wide and seven inches long as he pulled the staples.

"Don't try to take these off," he said. "They will come off on their own when it is time."

"Why are you skipping some of the staples?" I asked.

"They are not ready to be removed yet. I will take them out next week."

He finished this part of his work, and I left the room for the rest. In a short time, Linda was done, and we visited with the scheduler to get the plans for the weeks ahead. We also got other information on the chemo class we needed to take. Everyone at the Cancer Center was very good about keeping our spirits up, even though cancer was still new and confusing to us. We left the doctor's office and returned to the seats by the waterfall to sit and talk for a while.

LOOSE ENDS

I had a small job I was working on in my shop. I am fortunate enough to work at home just a few feet outside my back door. We have a cordless phone system so Linda could call me if she needed some help with anything. I checked on her about every thirty minutes anyway, but it was good to know she could reach me.

I worked for a while, and I saw our postman stop at our mailbox. We were waiting on a letter from DHS, so I walked out to the mailbox hoping to receive our letter. I grabbed the mail and was thumbing through it as I walked back to the house—electric bill, a sale at the grocery store, coupons, and a credit card application. What makes these people think I want their credit card? Then I saw the letter from DHS. I walked a little faster to the house to tell Linda.

"A letter from DHS!" I yelled as I stormed through the front door.

I tore the envelope open and removed the single piece of paper. I unfolded the paper and right on top were the words "Request denied." I sat down on the sofa next to Linda so she could see.

"This is what they told us would happen," I said.

We read a little further and the letter told us if we felt this was not correct or an error to call and set up an appointment with their review department. Linda took the letter and read the rest of it a few times and called the DHS number. She was only on the phone about two minutes after giving her name and case number.

"What did they say?" I asked as she hung up the phone.

"They said they would send another letter in a few days with an appointment time and date to see one of their counselors."

"We have a lot of appointments already. I hope it doesn't interfere with one of the others?"

"They said we could reschedule if we were unable to be there for the date they set."

"I'm just tired of telling all the doctor offices we are waiting on Medicaid. We already have bills from the hospital."

"Doesn't Jesus tell you not to worry?" she said.

"Yeah, He does. I wish it was that easy for me."

Linda has to remind me from time to time of the things I know. I thought about the verse that tells me that if worry can't even do a simple thing like add time to my life, then I need to wait on God (Luke 12:25-26). If adding time to life is a simple thing for God, then DHS is a very tiny problem for Christ to handle.

We also got another letter this same day that told us my own health insurance would be activated the first of the month. This did not seem too important at the time because I was healthy and had no medical needs.

I went back to work until it was time for me to fix lunch. This was a day that Marsha would be here to check Linda's blood pressure. *That's all she ever does*, I thought, *and we could do that for ourselves*. But she did answer a lot of our questions and always lifted Linda's spirit with her joyful attitude.

I fixed us a can of soup and a grilled cheese sandwich for lunch—nothing too exotic, but I was still learning. We had lunch, and Marsha pulled into our driveway when we were almost finished. I quickly put our plates in the kitchen and met her on the front porch.

"Hi Marsha, good to see you," I said and she handed me a pie. "What's this?"

"It's a caramel pecan," she said. "I told you I would make you a pie."

"Thank you. We just finished lunch. Would you like me to cut you a piece?"

"Oh, no thank you. I have another appointment at two o'clock, and I am trying not to be late."

She came in and went across the room to sit next to Linda.

"I've got pie," I said and took it to the kitchen.

When I returned, both of them were talking at the same time again, and I don't think they even noticed me. How do they do that? I mean talk and listen at the same time. I can ask Linda a question while she is watching the television and reading a book, and she will not miss a thing. I can lose track of everything if a fly lands on my arm.

I went to my office down the hall until Marsha was ready to leave. When the girls were done, I walked Marsha to her car as she talked all the way. I thanked her for the pie and hurried back in to test it.

The next few days were about the same. Linda took a lot of naps, I did laundry and dishes and sometimes some of the old work I use to do, like mow the yard. I think I was starting to get use to the extra work I had to do.

The weekend arrived and our good friends Ted and Cheryl, whom we met at church years ago, brought dinner over and shared the meal with us. Afterwards, Cheryl helped me clean up the kitchen, and the four us sat down to watch a Christian movie. They did not stay too much longer to keep from wearing Linda out. It was a great evening to spend with lifelong friends.

"Let's go out for breakfast," Linda said as we got out of bed Saturday morning.

"Are you up to it?"

"Yeah, I feel good. Then maybe we can go see one of the kids."

"Okay, whatever you want to do."

We went to the bathroom to get ready. The first thing we always did was drain the Foley. Then we needed to put on the leg bag. I got all the pieces we had rigged together a few weeks ago. I had only done this a few times, but it worked much smoother after that first time. I was about to unhook the big bag, but the tube was full and I could not get it to drain.

"I don't know what's keeping the tube from draining," I said. "I can't unhook it like this."

I shook and twisted the tube trying to get it to drain, but it would not. "This is a new problem," I said.

"I wish I could get rid of this thing."

"You will soon enough."

I opened a valve near the middle of the hose, but it didn't appear to help.

"Something is not right," she said.

"What?"

"The catheter is falling out."

It's a bit embarrassing; they really should give directions, but after an emergency trip to the hospital, I found out the valve I opened should not be touched. That valve is filled with saline for the purpose of keeping the catheter in.

Needless to say, we missed our breakfast. After repairs were made to my fumble, and they installed all new equipment, we left the hospital and had an early lunch instead of breakfast. Afterwards, we returned home.

I told Linda, "Dr. Kevin will probably enjoy this story Monday morning when we go to his office. I may be the world's first husband to accidently remove a catheter."

Our kids came over later that day. They got a good laugh about my mistake. Sometimes I think they like to see me mess up. The Sunday school class I teach is the same way. They also like to ridicule me with every opportunity I give them, and it doesn't take much. I did not tell them about this one.

Sunday morning we decided to stay home from church. Linda had more than enough to do Saturday with the catheter emergency, and I had someone filling in for me in my class while Linda was recovering from the surgery. Linda needed the rest anyway because we had a very big week ahead of us.

Monday, Dr. Kevin at the Cancer Center said Linda's bladder had healed enough to remove the catheter. He also removed the rest of the staples. What a great day that had become. Linda was free of all extra hardware except a few pieces of tape. He reminded us of the chemo class we were to take Wednesday evening. We could bring any friend or family member to the class that would be helping us as we go through the chemo. We got home late that afternoon and found the letter we were waiting on from DHS and I opened it.

"They have an appointment time for us at nine o'clock Thursday morning. Do we have anything else Thursday?" I asked.

"I don't think so..." Linda started searching for other events on her calendar.

"The letter says we will be seeing Don Williams. I thought he was a country singer."

"I'm sure it's not the same man," Linda said.

"I remember playing golf one day with MacGyver," I said. "And we used to square dance with Bob Hope."

None of these people were famous, but it made for good conversation if you were old enough to know the famous names.

Linda had already crashed on the sofa. It had been a long day for her, and she needed the rest.

"Help me get up," she said as she reached out to me.

"What do you need?"

"I have to go to the bathroom."

This was something new and different for us. This hadn't been taking place for over three weeks. This every-day activity that had been taken away had returned.

I remember when we first started building our house and our lives in the country where we live. We did not have running water for a while. I brought the water into our house in buckets I filled from other places. When we did get running water in our house, it did not take very long to take it for granted. Getting rid of the Foley bag was like getting rid of those buckets, but Linda had to get used to it.

Tuesday was without any scheduled plans, and I'm glad it was. I needed to get some of my work done and call a few of my customers. I manufacture tooling for foundries. That is getting harder to do because so much is now being done in other countries. I have some ideas on how to fix that problem, but the government hasn't called for my help yet. I have enough to deal with in my own house for now, so they will have to wait.

I spent the morning on the phone and in my e-mail. I quoted a few small jobs, but wondered when I might have time to do them. Marsha came by around ten in the morning and I stayed with my work. I never realized how much paperwork Linda did with the business and the personal files until she took the last two months off. I would be adding eight to ten hours work on top of the ten I added for cooking and cleaning each week.

By the end of the day there was still much to do, but you have to know how to stop. I warmed up some leftovers from the night before. We had dinner and decided everything else could wait until tomorrow. I had found out what it was like to be working three jobs, and I didn't want at least two of them but I had no choice.

On Wednesday, Linda reminded the kids that our chemo class was that night if they were able to come. We had been writing down our questions so we would not forget any of them. Chemo, just like cancer, felt like it was for someone else. Not for us. Would Linda lose her hair? How soon and how long would chemo last? What were some of the other side effects? Chemo is a frightening subject when we didn't even know what it was, but we are so fortunate to have others around to teach us and help us get through it.

I got a little more work done and caught up on a few more projects as the day went by. Linda was improving in her health every day, so we left a little early for the chemo class and stopped for dinner at a real restaurant. That's what Linda calls it when we are not at a fast food place. She says she likes to slow down and have a chance to chew her food. I am always in a hurry and could live on cheeseburgers. After thirty-five years of marriage, you have to wonder how we made it. I always finish my meal and look at Linda's plate still three quarters full. Sometimes I try to help her, but not always with success.

We arrived at the chemo class and met up with my daughter Leslie there. She informed us her church class would be providing a meal for us each Sunday afternoon for a while. God was finding so many ways to help us in our time of need, and I made plans to visit her class to share our story and to thank them personally.

We found our way to the room for the chemo class. Another couple and the instructor were already there.

"Hi. You must be Bob and Linda," the instructor said.

"Yes," I said. "And this is my daughter Leslie."

"Hello, Leslie, my name is Amy. I am glad to meet all of you. Linda, here is a book for you and your family to use tonight. You can take this home with you for quick reference, and here is a package of other gifts and information you can use later."

Shortly after another couple came in, Amy said, "Okay, we are all here for tonight so we can sit down and get started. Please feel free to eat any of the snacks in the back and the restrooms are just down the hall to the right. I am a nurse with Hillcrest hospital, and I have been working with cancer patients for twenty-one years. I know all of you have lots of questions, and I will ask you to hold them until the end. Most of your questions will be answered as we go through the blue cancer book you have already received."

We spent the next hour and a half going through our book. It started off with "What Is Chemotherapy" and ended with emergency phone numbers to call for any problems.

It covered different types of chemo (over a hundred), other medications, platelets, hair loss, neuropathy, cognitive dysfunction, and many other words we did not understand. It even had information on emotional changes and taste and smell changes. Any time you put a horde of chemicals in your body to kill cancer, changes take place in areas you don't want to change.

We listened to the instructor, we heard a few stories from the guests, and we asked our questions at the end. The class did answer a lot of questions, but it also raised a few we hadn't thought of. We gathered our things and returned to our cars in the parking lot.

"I'm not sure if I feel better or worse after all that. It was a lot to take in," I said.

"You know, now we have some answers," Linda said. "We know what to expect and we have places to call if we need help."

"We better start looking for a wig," I said.

"I want one that looks the same as it is now, so no one will know."

"I'm sure we can do that," I said as we pulled out of the parking lot.

We headed for home with more information, but no less uncertainty. There are a lot of problems we covered tonight that could come with the chemo. There could be new problems we didn't even think of, but we also know some of our worries will never happen. We were both glad we had this class to help us understand a little about what is coming up.

It was Thursday morning, the day of our meeting with Don Williams at the DHS office. We prayed about this meeting and asked for God's blessings on ourselves and on Don. We gathered all the paperwork and tax forms we were to bring with us. Most of them were still in the folder we put together a month ago.

We entered the DHS building through the metal detectors and went up to the second floor where we were the last time. The Christian lady we met when we were there before asked if she could help.

"Yes, we have a meeting this morning with Don Williams," I said.

She told us, "Go to the first floor. All counseling is downstairs."

They took our paper downstairs, and we sat in the waiting area with about fifty other people. When we were called in to Mr. Williams's office, we told him of our circumstances, lack of work, and lack of insurance. He took our last year's tax returns and this year's payroll and left the room for about twenty minutes.

Borrowing money is not always the best thing to do, but I felt like I did the first time I tried to get a loan for a car as a teenager. *I hope we get this. I hope we get this.* If we didn't get some help, I feared I would never reach the end of the hospital bills. I knew Linda was all that mattered, but I couldn't help feeling a little worried.

Don returned to his office and asked us a few more questions as he filled out our answers on his paper. Then he asked, "What is Social Security doing for you?"

That question surprised me. How did he know we had talked to Social Security?

Linda answered, "I have a phone meeting with them at two o'clock Monday. I was unable to go to their office because I was in the hospital that week."

"Okay, call me back when you find out what they are going to do. I think we will be able to help you out. It's good to be able to give help to someone that needs it."

"Does that mean you can help us?"

"I have to know what Social Security is going to do first. Call me as soon as you know."

We thanked him and left the building feeling a little better, but we still didn't know for sure if we were going to get the help we needed. To make things worse, we already had a lot of unpaid medical bills and still no solution. And the next day, Linda was getting a port put in. We had already received a $52,000 bill just from the hospital, and we are only getting started. That was more than our first house cost, and that house took twelve years to pay off.

The very next day, we returned to Hillcrest hospital to get the port put in. Once again they asked, "Who is your insurance carrier?"

They always accepted our answer, "We are waiting on Medicaid."

I am not sure how that helped, but they kept letting us in. I was sure that if Medicaid did not help soon, the hospital would be expecting us to pay.

The medical assistant explained what they were going to do. He showed us a medical drawing on the wall of a port and how it is connected to the artery coming out of the heart. He explained how this is better for chemo patients so the chemo does not do damage to the veins in your arms.

"How much does it cost?" I asked, knowing it was a stupid question.

"I really don't know," he said. "I just help the doctor with the procedure."

Linda asked the more intelligent questions. "How long will I be out?"

"We don't put you out at all; we just make you groggy so you don't care."

"How long can we leave the port in?" Linda asked.

"It can stay in for 10 or more years. Your doctor will let you know when it can be removed."

"Do I need to do anything with it?"

"No, it will be under your skin and you won't see it. There will be three small bumps you can feel with your finger. Those bumps are so the nurse will know where to place the needle for chemo and other treatments. The port will have to be flushed out about every six weeks by a medical facility with a saline solution." He paused and said, "Any other questions?"

I thought about the last time I had something to do with a saline solution, a catheter fell out, and so I kept my mouth shut.

Linda had no other questions, and the two of them left the room for the minor surgery. I found myself again in a waiting room. My mind wanders when it is alone and this time it took off wondering about the bills. *How much is this one? How much do we already owe? What is DHS going to do?* I know I should just let God do what He is going to do, but when I am alone,

I sometimes think without the help of the Holy Spirit. I opened my phone to call anyone, just to talk, but we were in the middle of the hospital, and I could not get a signal through so many walls. I pressed the Bible button on the side of my phone to let God talk to me in my time of need. It opened to where I left off a few days ago.

I had never believed opening the Bible would instantly speak to me, but that day it did. I read: "With man this is impossible, but not with God; all things are possible with God," found in Mark 10:27. I whispered, "Thank you, Jesus" and remembered He is with us always.

CHEMOTHERAPY STARTS

It was one minute until two o'clock when the phone rang. Social Security said they would call at two that afternoon, but I never thought they would be that punctual. We were waiting for the call even though we are not sure of what they could do to help us.

Linda went on and on giving vital information and doctor and hospital information, answering all their questions. Linda was taking notes and passing along the same data that we gave at DHS. She was on the phone for a full forty-five minutes.

Linda finally said "Thank you," and hung up the phone.

"Well, that was a full length meeting," I said.

She began weeping a little.

"No help from them I guess."

"No, they're going to help. They said due to the cancer and the surgery, I am disabled," Linda said.

"Well you haven't done any work for a few months," I said.

I had removed Linda from the payroll three months ago.

"They are going to give me a disability check each month and then review the disability in four to six years."

"Wow! How much are they going to give you?"

She pointed to the figure she had written down on the paper.

"Wow!" I said. "That's more than I have been paying you."

I didn't pay her very much and certainly not what she was worth.

Her weeping grew a little louder. "This will really help," she said.

"You never know what God is going to do. Call DHS and tell Don what Social Security said. I wonder if they will help since Social Security is helping. Maybe that's why he wanted to know."

Linda went through her notes looking for the DHS phone number and case number. She placed the call and was told that Mr. Williams would return her call around four o'clock.

I was looking at Linda's notes from Social Security when she hung up the phone.

"When will they send you this check?" I asked.

"They will do a direct deposit into the bank starting in August."

"I'm sorry, but I still can't believe it until I see it. I'm an old man, and I've never gotten this kind of help from anyone."

"That's what they told me."

"Did you get the name of the person you talked to or some account numbers or something?"

"Yes, it's all on that paper."

"Well, I think I will laminate this paper and put it in a frame. I will hang it in my office," I said, still not believing we could receive this help.

I jumped up and went to my office to plug the numbers into my spreadsheet to see how this would help by the end of the year. It was impossible to tell without all the expense data, but it felt good to put in some numbers that showed some promise. I ran everything on a spreadsheet in my computer, and I was still playing with the numbers when the phone rang. Most calls are for Linda so I let her get it. It wasn't long before she came to my office.

"Medicaid is going to help us with the medical bills all the way back to March," she said.

"Do you mean everything for the last two months?"

"Yes."

"The hospital bill?"

"And the doctors."

How do you describe the feeling you have when many thousands of dollars are forgiven? *Only God could make something like that happen*, I thought. That day, we received hope and light at the end of the tunnel.

We decided to celebrate so I took Linda to the wig store. We knew she would need a wig soon, and this was a good time. I didn't care what the wig might cost, I just wanted the best for my wife, and she was going to get it. They had real hair and synthetic hair.

"The real hair costs a little more," the store clerk said, "But it is also heavier and requires more work to take care of it."

Linda looked at both. I could not tell the difference without touching it. It wasn't too difficult to choose, Linda wanted something that looked like her real hair she had then. She found one that was close to identical.

"How does this one look?" Linda said.

"You look like you did when we left the house. Are you sure you don't want something different?"

"No, I like this one. How much is it?" she asked the clerk.

"It's seventy-eight dollars."

I was thinking they would be hundreds of dollars. "Wow," I said, "You can have that one and another if you want."

"No. I'll take this one," she said.

"Do you want to wear it or put it back in the box?" the clerk asked.

Linda looked in the mirror again and said, "I will wear it."

I paid the clerk and we left the store. When we got in the car Linda said, "Go to Leslie's house. I want to see if she will notice anything different."

Leslie lived only one mile away from where we were, so I drove to her house. If anyone was going to notice, it would have to be my daughter. I don't know anyone in the world who can spend as much time fixing hair as she does. Leslie would get up two hours before school to work on her hair. My other daughter was not to be disturbed until only five minutes remained before we had to leave. I never understood the hours of preparation. Both of my girls look good without accessories.

Leslie was in the front yard with her daughter when we arrived. Leslie and her mother talked for a good ten minutes. Linda finally gave in and had to ask, "Do you like my hair?"

"I thought it looked like you got some highlights. Who did it?"

"It's my new wig. What do you think?"

"That's a wig?" she said as she reached up to touch it. "I thought it looked a little different, but I thought you just got it fixed. It looks great."

Linda's day was made, without a doubt. She had Medicaid approval, Social Security disability payments, and now, most importantly, our daughter's approval on the wig and her granddaughter sitting in her lap.

We visited a little longer, and Linda wore her new wig the rest of the day even though she didn't need it. I had a very happy and content wife at the end of this day.

We don't usually set the alarm, but this morning, we needed to be at the hospital at eight for the first chemo treatment. Yes, we had a class, and we knew some things, but there was still the unknown. We found our way to the fifth floor and room number 527. It was a room no larger than our bedroom with six recliners. The nurse in the room turned and faced us.

"Hello Mary," I said as I read her name tag. "Is this where we come for chemo?"

"Yes. Which one of you will be getting the chemo?" Mary said.

"I wish I could do it for her, but Linda will be taking it."

"Okay Linda. Have a seat in one of the chairs, and I will go get your file."

Linda sat down, and I sat on a stool with wheels. I rolled over to her location and held her hand. Mary came back, opened a nearby drawer, and pulled out a sealed package. She tore it open and laid out the tools on a small table near the chair. It was full of tubes, needles, and gloves. She began taking Linda's blood pressure. "Is this your first chemo treatment?"

"Yes."

"Do you have a port?" she asked as she took a look for herself.

"Yes. It was put in about two weeks ago," Linda said.

"Good. That will make things much easier on you. We can do everything through this one connection."

As she was putting on her gloves, Mary told us she had ordered the two chemo types prescribed by the doctor, and they would be ready in about fifteen minutes. She found Linda's port and explained what she was going to do. She sprayed the spot with a painkiller and placed a needle coming out of a small piece of plastic into her port. A small tube extended out from the plastic about fourteen inches. She placed a clear patch of tape over the port area so the needle would not be moved for the rest of the day.

Another patient entered the room and sat down.

Mary attached a large syringe to the hose and pushed in a saline mixture for cleaning the port. Next, she drew out three large tubes of blood for test purposes. The first one was not used as it held most of the saline. "I will take these to the lab and will be back shortly."

When Mary came back, she hung three bags of clear liquid on the pole near Linda's chair.

"We will begin putting this in when I get the report back from the lab. We have to make sure your blood counts are high enough for the chemo before we start."

"How long does this take?" I asked.

"This first one will take about seven hours. We will put it in really slow the first hour to make sure Linda does not have an allergic reaction. We will be able to put it in the next time in five to six hours."

Mary began doing the same procedure to the other patient as a few more came in. She was in and out of the room taking care of four patients. She came back to Linda and said, "Your blood counts look good," and she started her chemo.

It's really not much of a spectator's event after this. Once the IV has started, we just sat around and waited. They had snacks and drinks for the patients, and they would be serving lunch. After the first hour had passed, Mary increased the flow rate of the chemo treatment going into my wife.

Linda had her books to read and people to talk to, so I left and returned at three that afternoon. I did the grocery shopping, returned home and put the groceries away. I quoted another small job that I found in my fax machine, and by then it was time to head back to the hospital.

When I arrived, Linda was on the last bag of chemo. "Looks like you're almost done," I said.

Mary was there and she heard me. "No, I have to run a small bag of saline through after that one," she said. "It will take another thirty minutes."

"Okay," I said and sat down next to Linda. "How are you feeling?"

"Everything is fine. I feel the same as I did this morning."

"You still have hair," I said joking with her.

"For now," Linda said. "Mary told me it may not start falling out until the next chemo treatment in three weeks. She said I will get real tired and sleepy in a few days too."

"Oh you're just trying to get out of cooking and stuff."

"I wish I felt like cooking or doing anything."

"We will get there. God is in control," I said.

Linda introduced me to Becky across the room. "Becky had this chemo treatment seven years ago, and now she is doing it again. Her cancer came back."

"I'm sorry to hear that Becky," I told her, "A person should not have this once, and you have had to do it twice."

"Yes, and I hope this is the last time. I have a friend that has had cancer seven different times."

"That is just not right," I said.

Linda said, "Tom was in here this morning, and he has to take radiation once a week with his chemo."

"I hope you got everybody's name so we can put them on our prayer list at church," I said.

We talked until the last of the saline was used up. Then Linda was disconnected, and we were on our way. Sometimes we think we are in a bad way, but we can always find someone fighting a bigger problem. It's not easy to feel good about having cancer, but there are many worse things to have.

"I have to come back in here every Thursday until the chemo is done," Linda said when we got in the car.

"How come? I thought this was every three weeks."

"They have to draw blood every week."

"Okay. They're close to home, and we have Medicaid now. We can be thankful for both of those."

Linda laid her seat back a few inches, closed her eyes and said, "Let's go home."

Thursdays would be our big day of the week; one for chemo, one for blood work, and the third for blood work and a visit at the Cancer Center with Dr. Kevin. Then we would start all over again.

Marsha came by for her last visit on Friday. The weekly visits to the hospital would replace the home care that we needed. Marsha would be missed, and Linda told her she could stop by for a visit anytime.

Saturday, we went for a walk at the mall. Linda was getting stronger as she healed from the surgery. Sunday was our first lesson on what the chemo treatments do to the body. Sunday, and for the next two or three days after chemo, Linda would be too tired and depressed to do anything. This was the routine we were about to follow for every chemo treatment. Not only did the chemo make Linda feel bad, but it would also keep her from sleeping.

The next Wednesday, we received the Medicaid card we needed in the mail. That made all the future visits to the doctor and the hospital a lot easier, and we only had to pay a small co-pay amount.

We went about our new routines of life for the next few weeks. Whatever life brings to you, you begin to live that way and treat it as normal, but cancer is not normal. Life had already been disrupted with surgery, worry, and many other unknowns. Now we would have to learn the effects of the chemo chemicals on Linda's body. The new surprises of each day were becoming the new "normal" for us.

A few days after the second chemo treatment, Linda came into my office where I was working. "My hair is falling out," she said.

I turned and looked at her. "It looks fine to me."

Linda pulled on her hair and a small handful came out. "It's time to get it cut," she said. "I don't want it all over my house."

We had already talked to my uncle who is also my barber. He has been cutting hair for about thirty years. He told us to call on the day we needed to cut Linda's hair, so I placed the call I had been dreading.

I got off the phone and told Linda he said to come over at five o'clock. We could do this after hours when no one was there.

"We knew this was going to happen," Linda said.

"I know. It's just not your usual hair cut. I knew I was going to get a root canal once, but I wasn't looking forward to it."

"I have my wig."

"I know. And it looks good."

Linda was more ready than I was. I think if it was my hair being lost, I wouldn't care. Bald men are everywhere. I quickly calculated that, in three-and-a-half months, chemo would be over, and she could grow her hair back. After all, I raised my kids for twenty years and that didn't seem to take very long.

We got to the barber shop. Uncle Finis put up the closed sign and locked the door after we came in. Linda sat in the barber's chair.

"I know you have done this a few times," I said.

My nephew had cancer and chemo ten years ago. He was twenty-seven when cancer took his life. Uncle Finis had removed his hair also.

"Yes, I have," he said. "In thirty years a lot of my customers have had to lose their hair. The hardest ones are family."

He reached for his clippers and faced Linda to go to work. I could see a tear in his eye and that put one in mine as well. It was not easy for me to watch, but I think it was even harder to do. *It has to be the hardest when it's a woman*, I thought. But Linda was doing well with her back to the mirrors.

When Uncle Finis was finished, I handed Linda her wig. She and my uncle's wife, Phyllis, put it on her head. Phyllis adjusted the wig and brushed it a little. Then, for the first time, Linda turned and faced the mirror. She still had not seen what the rest of us had seen, and probably would not until later tonight. She and Phyllis adjusted and fixed the wig to her liking. You could not tell it wasn't her own hair.

I remembered when my hair was cut off in boot camp many years ago. My hair was longer and thicker than Linda's, and when I looked in the mirror, I was shocked and felt naked. I knew Linda would see her head later, and I wished she didn't have to.

"I think that was harder on you two than it was on me," she said.

"It wasn't the best part of my day," I said.

"I have been preparing for this for weeks. I know it has to be this way, and I am ready. It's just hair, it will come back."

Uncle Finis said, "This is never easy, no matter how many times I do it."

We thanked him and returned home. Linda wore her wig until bedtime. I didn't think she wanted to look under her wig, but when she did I could tell she had accepted being bald weeks ago. She has a good dozen hats to wear, and she picked one that would keep her warm at night and put it on. I was still discouraged about the hair loss, but Linda seemed to handle it okay. It took only a few more days for the eyelashes and eyebrows to fall out also. That turned out to be the hardest part for her.

For the next few weeks Linda only wore her wig when we left the house. Around the house, she wore a hat or tied a scarf around her head. We learned to accept the bald head as a trophy. "It signifies, 'I am a cancer survivor.'" Linda and I both learned to have little regard for hair. It is life that counts. It wasn't long before Linda would wear her wig only to church. Anyplace else didn't matter.

In the weeks to follow, the grandkids learned to pull off whatever Grandma was wearing on her head. They liked to run their little hands over her head and feel the nubbies. That's what our oldest granddaughter of three named them—nubbies.

Our second oldest granddaughter, almost three, liked to wear a scarf tied on her head just like Grandma. It would fall off several times a day, but she would put it right back on. Sometimes she had it on backwards or inside out, but she was proud to be like Grandma. It made Grandma feel good, and it showed us how unimportant hair really is.

Sometime after the third chemo treatment, Linda attended a class to learn how to use makeup when you have no hair. When she painted on her eyebrows they were not always even. One side would look normal and the other side would look surprised. There are many classes to help cancer patients, and this free class gave her around a hundred dollars worth of makeup and taught her how to put on eyebrows when you have no guide lines.

Linda had received her fourth chemo treatment, and it was like the others. Linda always became tired, depressed, and very emotional. For four or five days Linda didn't leave the house. She felt worthless and nothing I did or said seemed to be of any value. She was tired but couldn't sleep. She was bored and couldn't read or watch the television. She loves to work in her garden, but couldn't be in the heat or the dirt. As more treatments were received, the results seemed to get worse.

The other side effects were tingling fingers and toes. Her feet felt like they were asleep all the time. She had at least one arm or one leg that was in a tapping motion all day long. It was a miserable few days for both of us. It made me sad because I could do nothing about it. It hurt me to see Linda hurt. This was something I could not fix, and we soon had a new side effect.

"Look at my eye!" she yelled.

I looked and all of the white part on her right eye had turned bright red as if it were bleeding.

"Did you poke it or something?" I asked.

"No. What's wrong with it?"

If it had not been one of the chemo emotional days, she might not have been so upset, but I didn't know what was wrong either. I did, however, stay calm in the face of alarm, but that too, was a put on.

"Let's call the Cancer Center and see what they say. They will tell us what to do."

Linda had calmed down just a little because I was calm (you can fool some people some of the time). Linda called the Cancer Center. She knew almost everyone over there by name and knew who to talk to. The five minutes she was on the phone caused her to calm down even more.

"What did they say?" I asked.

"They said it is a common problem. Sometimes a tiny blood vessel in the eye will break and the eye fills with blood. They said as long as there is no leakage or pain, it will most likely go away in about three days."

"Do they want you to come in?"

"No. Not unless it gets worse."

"Well, did you tell them we'll keep an eye on it?" I laughed, trying to make her feel better.

"It scared me," she said, weeping.

"I was as scared as you were. I was just trying to keep you calm."

By the end of the day, about ten percent of her eye had returned to normal. That's not much, but it was getting better. By noon the next day about half of the red had gone away, and in three days, it was gone like they said.

There are a lot of side effects with chemo and the other nine drugs she was taking with the chemo. I looked at the side effects on aspirin one time and decided to keep the headache; it wasn't half as scary as what could happen.

I am not very good about taking a pill for anything. How do I know if I am getting better if my sickness is covered up with drugs? However, when I am sick enough, I thank God that he provided doctors who are smart enough to help us through it as God heals us

> He forgives all my sins and heals all my diseases.
>
> Psalms 103:3 NLT

THE LAST CHEMOTHERAPY

We were walking out of Hillcrest hospital. Linda had just received her fifth chemo treatment with one more to go. We watched a man quickly pull into a handicap parking space, jump out of his car, and run for the hospital door.

"Hey, you forgot your crutches," I yelled at him.

He waved at me with one finger (to prove his intelligence) and disappeared.

"Don't worry about it," Linda said.

"But he is stealing from someone else in need. Why does he think he is better than a man with no legs that might be driving by? It just makes me mad. You remember when your legs were broken and how many times I had to park a quarter mile away?"

"I remember."

Linda is not authorized for handicap parking with her cancer, but she was when both of her legs were broken. At that time, we had another very intelligent person park against our car while we were in a handicap space. When I brought Linda back to the car in her wheelchair, I could not get her in the car. Some idiot had parked where there wasn't even a parking space. I had to move our car to get Linda in.

I see people abusing this parking space all the time and others parking where there is no space at all. I have seen people with a walker park twenty spaces away because the handicap spaces were full of unjust users. I can't turn the cars over or flatten their tires as my rebellious nature wants to do, but I can do something else Jesus taught us to do, and Linda has to remind me of that more than I care to admit. We can pray for them.

> But I say, love your enemies! Pray for those who persecute you!
>
> Matthew 5:44 NLT

"Let's go eat," I said in frustration.

"I need to go to the drug store and pick up three prescriptions," Linda said.

"Okay. There are a lot of places to eat over there. Where do you want to go?"

That was really a stupid question. We play this game with most meals. Another side effect of chemo is that you can't taste anything.

"It doesn't make any difference, you pick something," she said.

"How about Mexican? You said you could taste that sometimes."

"I don't want Mexican."

"Okay, that's why I asked you what you want."

"Don't make me decide. I can't do that right now."

I just shut up and drove to the drug store, hoping the face I was making in my mind didn't find its way out. The chemo poison in her body was playing games with her brain again. It is good for killing the cancer, but it pushes out all the hair and weakens other organs and sometimes the brain gets a little confused—hers and mine.

By the time we had finished at the drug store, Linda and I both had calmed down to reasonable, but I still picked a place to go eat. Some of the time, I don't ask where to go. I just park the car and ask if this is okay. This time it was.

Linda loves working in her garden, so after lunch she wanted to go somewhere to look at plants. I took her to a large hardware store. Many times when we shop, Linda goes her way and I go mine. Today was no different.

I went to the tool department to see if they had any tools I didn't already own. I have been in business a long time, and I use tools this hardware store has never heard of. I found nothing this trip and returned to the garden area where I left Linda. I found her in the outside part of the store talking to strangers. This is not unusual because Linda meets new people all the time. I walked over and stood next to her.

"This is my husband Bob," she told the couple.

"Hi."

"Hi. I noticed your wife's hat," the lady said, "and I thought she might be a cancer victim. I had a hat like that when I had cancer."

We talked with this couple for three or four minutes, and then Linda leaned on me pretty hard. I faced her and caught her as she began dropping to the floor. I sat her down on the cement and asked someone to get some help. Linda was only out for a few seconds.

"I think I got too hot," she said.

She was sitting between my legs, leaning against me. "Just sit here. I have some help coming," I told her.

We were only twenty yards from the outside checkout area. The girl from the checkout carried an umbrella over and used it to put Linda in the shade. She also handed me a bottle of cold water. I opened it and gave it to Linda.

"Drink some of this," I told her.

We sat on the floor for about five minutes. More help from the store had arrived to see if we were all right.

"Do you want us to call an ambulance?" someone asked.

"No, I'll be all right," Linda said.

The summer heat had arrived, and we did not realize Linda could not take the heat as she did before chemo. I had found one more thing to watch out for. When she was ready, we walked to the car and went home. After that I would check on her every few minutes when she worked in her garden.

Linda's four or five days of distress after chemo were coming to an end. We got a call from our church that Michelle had gone into the hospital. Michelle is a cute and happy little twelve year old who is a joy to be around. She was having trouble with passing out.

Linda got the call, and when she hung up the phone, she said, "Michelle from church has been in the hospital for two days. We need to go see her."

"Okay," I said. "What's wrong with her?"

"They don't know yet. Let's stop at the dollar store and get a bucket of snacks for them like we got from our Sunday school class."

"Yeah, that sounds like fun."

We went right to the dollar store. Everything we needed was there, including the bucket. We found the biggest one-dollar bucket in the store and used it for our shopping basket. We got cookies, chips, candy, and other junk. Just in case someone could not have all this sugar, we got a few healthy items too. We even added a coloring book and crayons.

It felt good to check out of the store doing something for someone else. So many good things had been done for us these last few months; it was great to get a chance to give something back.

We found Michelle's room at the hospital and carried the bucket into the room. We thought shopping for her was exciting, but that was nothing compared to Michelle going through this bucket while she was sitting in the middle of her bed.

"This is for you and your guests," Linda told her.

"I'm going to eat all this myself," she said as she pulled the bucket closer.

I laughed and told her mom, "I had the same reaction a few months ago when Linda and I received a bucket."

We sat down and talked to her mother as we watched her explore the highlight of her day. Michelle colored a picture for us of Jonah inside of a big fish. She returned home two days later.

Sunday morning, we got up to go to my daughter's church. Her Sunday school class had given us some help when Linda was in the hospital. I had made arrangements with her class to come in and give a report. I have been teaching for about ten years, and I was looking forward to this. I was going to have the whole hour to talk to them.

We had been to their church a half-dozen times before, but never to their class. We arrived a little early. It is a habit that I look over my notes one more time before class starts, only that day I had no notes because we had been living the story I was about to tell. We watched the class grow as the room filled up. All of the occupants were close to my daughter's age. Three of the couples had new born babies too young to leave in the nursery.

When it was time for class to begin, the usual teacher began taking prayer requests. The class had fifty-two people in it, counting the three babies. We attend a smaller church, and my average class size is about twenty. I have talked to our whole church a few times of about two hundred, but I knew them. This group I didn't know, and I found myself getting a little nervous.

We listened to the prayer requests and something happened that almost always happens with prayer requests. We heard the problems of others who I would not want to trade places with. Jesus said the poor would always be among you (Matt. 26:11). I think He was saying we would always have someone around needing help. I thought a person could be poor in money or in spirit and sometimes in health. Most of us are likely to experience all three. I paused for a moment to thank Jesus that our problems are small and that He was in control.

We prayed together and the instructor told the class of a few upcoming events and introduced me to the class. I took a place where all could see me. I have talked to many people many times, but this time my mouth went dry. I could feel my tongue sticking to the roof of my mouth.

"Good morning," I said. "This is my wife Linda," I pointed to her, "and by the grace of God, she is recovering from cancer," I smiled at her. "I am sure you all know my daughter Leslie," I pointed to her. "She and her husband brought to us at the hospital the collection you took up to help us. Linda and I wanted to thank you for the four dollars and thirty-five cents and the cheeseburger."

The class laughed and woke one of the babies.

"This class helped us a great deal, and I wanted to give you a full report," I continued. "I also would like to ask someone to tell me when my time is about over or I may talk all day." Someone raised their hand. "Thank you. First let me tell you about CA125. CA stands for cancer antigen. This number counts how many cancer cells are in the blood. When Linda started with the first chemo her number was at ninety-two. Anything below twenty-four is a good number, and today she is a nine."

The class responded with, "All right, way to go."

"Linda has one more chemo treatment to go, but we believe the cancer is already gone. Her last treatment is this next Thursday."

The class cheered, and I continued to explain the surgery and the results of the surgery and the hospital stay. Then we covered the chemo treatments, the frequency and the side effects, the many drugs needed to offset the chemo drugs and the blood test, hair loss, mood changes, and many of the other details.

Someone in the class asked, "Why would cancer come on so many people?"

"You have to understand who Satan is. He was once full of wisdom and beauty (Ezekiel 28:12), and he lived with God and was guardian of much (Ezekiel 28:14). Satan then became wicked, wanting to be more than his Creator (Ezekiel 28:15, Isaiah 14:14). God threw him out of heaven and down to the earth (Isaiah 14:12). Because of this, Satan hates God. To make it worse, God created man in His own image and put mankind in charge of all the earth (Gen. 1:26). Satan used to be in charge of much in heaven, and now he is not even in charge of this little earth. He knows God loves mankind. Satan wants to kill us in revenge and hatred toward God (1 Peter 5:8). You are of no importance to Satan, he doesn't want you, and he doesn't care about you. He only wants to hurt God."

I glanced at my daughter across the room. "Our family came to realize during surgery that Linda could have lost her life. Any one of us could be lost at any time and this made us see how important each of us is, not just to God, but to each other. God gave Linda some gifts to use in our family and other gifts to use in our church. Satan wants to kill all people and he doesn't care if they go to heaven or hell. He wants to kill because he hates God, and if the person is a Christian that will influence other people, then Satan wants to destroy them even more. Linda has influence on others, and she will for as long as she lives. Little did Satan know (he is not real smart) that so many people would be influenced by Linda over the months and years ahead. Because of her reactions and attitude toward the cancer and the treatment, many people will see what a Christ-filled person should look like. Satan's evil work will only draw others that are watching closer to Christ."

Someone stated, "It sounds like you will be attacked if you are a Christian."

"Yes you will be attacked. Jesus said, 'All men will hate you because of me' (Matthew 10:22). If unbelieving men will hate you, it is certain Satan will hate you. Look up the word persecuted in your Bible; you will learn much on this. The apostle Paul said in 2 Timothy 3:12, 'Everyone who wants to live a Godly life in Jesus Christ will be persecuted.' I had a man at work watching me for years just to point out errors in my Christian life. I told him to follow Jesus, not me. Persecution happens, and in this country, it is light. Jesus said you are blessed when people insult and persecute you because of Him (Matt. 5:11). The apostle James said to consider it pure joy (James 1:2)."

"But why does God allow bad things to happen?" someone asked.

"God gets the blame for everything. Insurance says they won't pay if it is an act of God. People ask 'Why did God take my son?' or 'Why did God allow this rape?' When we learn God's word, we can see He doesn't allow these bad things to happen, we do. God gave us a complete set of instructions for a wonderful life, but we chose not to follow Him (Romans 3:10, Prov. 20:9) and when bad things do happen, there will be a price to pay. If God were to hit each of us with a bolt of lightning when we sin, there would be no one on earth to strike because we have all broken God's standards (James 2:10). It is impossible for God to lie (Titus 1:2 NLT), and He gave the earth to us to rule (Gen. 1:28) until the end. God cannot say He has changed His mind and take back His word. Look at it this way. If someone is killed on the highway by a drunk driver, it was not God that took their life. It is not God that breaks into a house and shoots someone with a gun. Bad choices by others can take the life of someone else that has done nothing wrong. Our own bad choices can also take our life. No one makes us smoke or eat nothing but bad foods. The drugs a mother has taken may affect a baby at birth. It would be hard to answer why the life of a healthy baby is taken or why Linda has cancer, but it is not from God. He wants none to perish (2 Peter 3:9)."

The person watching the clock for me informed me my time was short, and I finished up. "Our struggle is not with our precious and wonderful God, it is against Satan (Eph. 6:12) and against the curse on the earth by our own sinful nature (Gen. 3:17 NLT). Satan will always continue to attack, so we must always keep the armor on that God has given us (Eph. 6:11). That armor is a six-piece set. Don't put on just the helmet and not the footgear. You may get shot in the foot. Load your sword with all the truth you can from God's word and you will not be taken down with Satan's lies. Remember God loves you (1 John 4:11) and your sins are forgiven (1 John 2:2)."

I closed with a prayer and took my seat. The dry mouth I started with stayed with me all the way through. As soon as I sat down, I was fine. We stayed after class for about twenty minutes to answer questions. We received a report later that the class really enjoyed our visit and would like for us to come back.

We got up early on Thursday. It had been four-and-a-half months since Linda's surgery. She was unable to drive the first two months, and I wouldn't let her drive with the chemo influence.

"This is it—the last treatment," I told her.

"I hope so. The doctor said I may need two more if the CAT scan shows anything still there. That test is two weeks away."

"Stop worrying about it. I know the cancer is gone."

"I'm not worried. I know I'm healed; I just want to see it on the test."

"I guess I do too, but it doesn't matter what the doctor says. What counts is what God says."

"It doesn't matter if this is the last one or not, I know the cancer will be gone."

"Is gone," I corrected her.

I remembered some friends we have who are sick all the time. I think it is because they say how bad things are before they happen. Our words have the power to move mountains (Matthew 17:20), and it is easy to call bad times on ourselves. If a person says nothing good ever happens to me, they are likely to get just that.

We headed for the hospital, and I walked Linda to the room as I always do each week. She sat in her favorite recliner, and Mary started her chemo routine. She always took Linda's blood pressure, and sometimes she would take mine. She didn't have to do this, but she knew mine was a little high, and she liked to check on me.

"Did you quit using so much salt like I told you?" Mary asked.

"No. I like salt,"

"You have to do something. Your blood pressure is way too high."

"I have an appointment with my doctor in three weeks."

"Good. You need to be around to take care of Linda," she said.

"Yes, but it's your turn to take care of Linda today. I have to go play golf or something. So I leave her in your wonderful hands."

I kissed Linda and before I left, I told her, "This is the last treatment."

She whispered, "Thank you, Jesus."

ANOTHER ATTACK

Linda met a new person at her last chemo treatment that told her of a cancer support group. Linda was invited to join the group. They met once a month for lunch to swap stories, information, and anything else they wanted to. Sometimes a special speaker would be there. Linda loves to be around people and was very excited to go. The first meeting for Linda was on Saturday on the other side of town. I hate to drive in all that traffic, and I've had to take her everywhere.

I told Linda, "You are over the surgery pain, the cancer is gone, and it has been nine days since your last chemo. I think you can drive. What do you think?"

"I think I can."

"Take your phone and call me when you get there, when you leave, and if you need me to come get you. Don't drive if you don't feel right."

"I'll be fine."

Linda had her car back and could go see the kids, shop, and go as she pleased. She drove to the support group and came home with many cancer stories with good endings. Cancer is still a horrible and scary disease, but it is not as deadly as it used to be. Many people have had cancer two or three times. One woman from our church had cancer seven times, and seven times she was cured. Linda shared a few stories with me from her two-and-a-half hour lunch and then she took a nap.

Three weeks had passed, and it was time for Linda's doctor visit. She had the CAT scan last week, and now it is time for us to get the results. I took her to the Cancer Center as I have done many times the last five months. She could drive herself, but I wanted to be with her for this report.

Dr. Kevin came into the examination room with his clipboard and took a seat on the short stool on wheels. He browsed through his papers one last time and looked up at us. "Your cancer is gone," he said.

Linda and I looked at each other. "You are healed," I said.

A look of joy and great excitement was on her face. We had been saying God was healing her from the day we learned about the cancer invading her body. We always believed the cancer would be taken away, and now it has been verified. We were both in high spirits with the report, and it was a real pleasure to see Linda's reaction to the news.

Dr. Kevin told us of a research test program he would like for Linda to take part in. It is for ovarian cancer survivors only. The purpose of the research study was to see if continued chemo might reduce the return of this type of cancer. It would mean she would be tested for cancer once a month, or continue chemo for once a month at a reduced amount. This test would last for one year, and we did not know if Linda would get the chemo or the cancer test until the research group made their decision.

I returned to the waiting area while the doctor finished with the exam. When Linda was finished, we went to another office where we could get more information about the clinical research program.

We learned that if Linda gets the observation part of the test, there would be little for her to do or think about. There would be blood tests, CAT scans once in a while, and little else. If she gets the reduced chemo, it would mean five or six hours a month receiving chemo just like she had been doing and staying bald for another year.

"You are already healed," I told her.

"Yes, but it might help others from having it a second time," Linda said. "And I would know it is not back in me again."

"I know you are always thinking of others. Whatever you decide to do, I will support you. I guess I was thinking of your hair."

"I have my wig if I need it. It is just hair, and I might not get the chemo."

"Okay. If you want this, so do I."

I didn't say anything else. It was her decision. I was thinking about her hair and not the good that might come from this research. Linda had already learned that hair was not that important. I wanted it back more than she did. I didn't want it for myself, but for her complete recovery. We saw her bald head as a survivor's trophy, but to cover that trophy with hair would be completion.

Linda did decide to take part in the research program, so we filled out all the questions and other information the research team wanted. We were done by noon. I still wasn't sure how I felt about this, but I also thought that if we wanted, we could stop anytime. That helped me a little, and Linda seemed pleased to be involved in research that might help someone else.

"You want to go someplace to eat?" I asked her. We don't eat out as often as we use to because of the reduced income.

"I want to go someplace nice," she said. "How about the Delta?"

"That works for me."

"Then I want to go buy some flowers for Mary at the hospital."

"Okay, how come?"

"She took good care of me, and I want to tell her thanks."

We stopped at the Delta Café and had lunch. Linda had some kind of fancy salad, and I had meatloaf. Linda has lots of books saying cancer patients should not eat red meat, but it is difficult for me to cut back. After all, I don't have cancer.

When we were done with lunch, we went flower shopping. Mary likes to work in the garden and so does Linda. We got something that was red and blue and green. It had little flowers and tiny peppers that were yellow and orange. I don't know anything about plants. I garden with the lawn mower.

We took the plant to Mary at the hospital. She was excited to see us and to receive a gift. Linda and Mary visited between patient calls, and I tried to stay out of the way. As we were leaving, Mary gave me a final warning about using too much salt.

Life started getting back to normal. Linda would cook a little more, and I did miss her cooking. She is much better at cooking than I am. She attended the cancer support group every month. The research program at the Cancer Center chose to check for cancer only—no additional chemo treatments. I was glad because if anything ever came up, I knew it would be caught early. And since she was not taking chemo, her hair had started growing back. I had not seen its true color for fifteen years because it was always colored. It was coming in dark brown and spotted with forty percent gray.

At Linda's last support group meeting, she discovered a man that had been bald for twenty-two years. After his chemo treatments, new life was brought to his bald head, and he grew hair. I would not recommend chemo as a hair treatment, and I don't know how long it lasted, but he grew hair.

There are many cancer groups of many different kinds, and Linda was taking part in several. One of them was the cancer survivors' walk. For our first event, we gathered at the River Parks. All of our kids and grandkids came with us. We had a free barbeque dinner, drinks, and entertainment. There were children dance groups and a country band that played a little rock and roll for us. The kids had a large playground. Linda and a few hundred others were given a pink T-shirt that said, "I am a cancer survivor." They were pink because this event was for the breast cancer survivors.

The survivor walk was only a half mile around some marked trees and a pink cancer car. All of our family made this little walk. Grandma Linda and our oldest granddaughter made another lap while the rest of us got things ready to go home. The walking would continue for twenty-four hours for anyone who wanted to support the walk against cancer.

It is a wonderful thing to be around survivors and to know you can beat this terrible disease. Cancer took a small chunk of time out of lives and the lives of other family members, but it did not win.

By the time November came around, Linda no longer wore her hats or her wig. She didn't have very long hair, but it was hers. It was curly (something she'd never had), and it was a little more gray. She wore it as a crown. It shows that she had cancer, and she has it no more. A few people at church thought Linda had gotten a haircut. Some of them did not even know of this cancer battle, and some didn't know she'd lost her hair.

When Christmas came around, we had much to thank the Lord for this year. We don't wait until the end of the year to say thank you to Jesus, but this Christmas brought the family together. We all still had each other, and we were thankful. I don't think there had been one day when Linda and our girls have not talked on the phone.

When it was March again, Linda celebrated her birthday and had enough hair to go get a trim but decided to wait until the next week. She also had her monthly visit to Dr. Kevin at the Cancer Center. I'd quit going with her a long time ago. When she returned home, she was not the same person who left the house that morning.

"What's wrong?" I asked her.

"The cancer is back. My CA125 is up to fifty-eight."

"What do you mean it's back? How can it be back?"

"I have ten or twelve small tumors around my uterus area," she said.

I thought about that for a moment and said, "It can't be too bad. They have been checking you every month."

"The doctor said they are too small to operate on, so he wants to start chemo again."

"Well, it can't be as bad as last time. Maybe the chemo will be a smaller amount."

"No, he said he wants to do the same thing as last time—six treatments, three weeks apart each time."

I sat down with a word on my mind that Christians try not to use. I'm not sure if that word came out or not. "Are you going to lose your hair again?" I asked.

"Yes."

The thought of that bad word came again. "You were about to go get a haircut," I said.

"This will save you twenty-five dollars."

"Help me find the good side," I said.

"We still have Medicaid."

"Okay, that's one."

"I still have my port, and there's no surgery."

"Yeah, that was a nightmare. When are they going to start?"

"In about three weeks," she said.

"How do you feel about this? I mean, I know how I feel," I said with discouragement.

"I've had a little more time to process this. I'll be okay."

"I know you will. It's just not right to start all over."

"This is why I wanted to be in the research program, in case there was something more," she said.

"That program was only open for thirty days. I guess God opened another door for us that we didn't see at the time."

Satan threw another punch, but we knew he was not going to win. Last year, Linda had surgery on April first. This year, she started chemo all over again on the same day—April first. But this time, she was healthier and we knew what to expect. The chemo days are still on Thursdays just like the last time, but this time, they are at the Cancer Center instead of Hillcrest—three times as far to drive.

The next week Dr. Kevin wanted to put Linda on a different research program. This one was a new drug that might help destroy the cancer. We didn't know if she would be getting the drug or part of the drug; it was a blind test. She wanted to be a part of the test to help someone else in the future.

"Is this what you want to do?" I asked her.

"Yes. I want to get rid of this cancer and I think this will help."

I placed my hands on her shoulders and prayed against the cancer and for the doctors involved and the new medication.

It had been a wonderful seven months without chemo. Now we had started again. The first treatment brought back the memories we would like to never remember. The five days after each chemo treatment brought fatigue, tingling in the toes and fingers, loss of taste, and sometimes a little depression.

To help with the despair at the end of the five days of gloom, we went to get Linda another wig. She was going to lose her hair again, so I thought she should have two hairdos. She got one about the same color, but a different style.

After the five days of gloom from the second treatment, we did have to go and cut off her newly received curly hair. I think this time it bothered her a little more than the first time. The new test drugs were being administered without any problem, but we weren't sure if she was really taking the drug or not.

The third and the fourth treatments seemed to bring more depression and worry to Linda than the first time through the treatments last year. I think most of it was because she didn't want this a second time. I didn't either, and I'm sure no one does.

We watched the numbers from the CA125 test each week coming down. It is now at twenty-three and the staff at the Cancer Center thinks Linda might be on the new test drugs, but no one can know for sure. We are just glad the cancer count is coming down fast.

We did get another shocking surprise just before the fifth chemo treatment. Here we are near the end of the second battle with cancer, and we got a letter from Medicaid. They decided to cancel the help they were providing at the end of that month. Three weeks from that day they would no longer help us.

Linda called Mr. Don Williams to find out what had happened. He was not available, but Linda left all the information she could and our need for help on the answering device.

"If you remember, last year we were denied their help until we had a meeting," I told Linda.

"I know, but I have one more chemo next month, and Dr. Kevin said he might want to do two more after that."

"I wouldn't worry about it too much. God carried us through this last year, and He isn't going to stop. He isn't going to leave us."

Linda tried to contact Mr. Williams a few times. It was almost a week before he called Linda back. He said he had gotten Linda's message and was talking to many people trying to get the Medicaid reinstated. He could not do it.

"What am I to do?" Linda asked him on the phone. "I have more chemo, and more tests, and we are close to being finished."

"I know you need this, and I have talked to everyone to reinstate it, but the answer is no. You can file a report in this office that will allow you to continue using the

Medicaid insurance, but in six or eight weeks there will be a hearing to see if you qualify. If you do not qualify, you have to pay back all the money spent after the first of the month plus other fees and penalties."

Linda said, "I will have to talk to my husband to see what we will do."

We were sitting at the dining room table going over the phone conversation. It seemed we would either not have Medicaid anymore or we risked paying for everything plus penalties (like a credit card company).

"What are we going to do?" Linda said through eyes full of tears.

"Well, we are not going to fight the government, and God is certainly wiser than they are (1 Corinthians 3:19). Let's step into my office for a minute," I said.

I opened a computer file with my contacts and phone numbers and called my insurance provider. We got approval for my insurance about the same time Medicaid started. I gave them my name and policy numbers and the call was forwarded to a woman named Amanda.

"I need to add my wife to this policy with a preexisting cancer condition. Would that be a problem?" I asked.

Amanda said, "No it looks like she was approved a year ago and we can just add her back on. It also looks like she was removed because Medicaid was being used."

"Yes. Medicaid just canceled us," I said.

"Do you have access to the internet and a fax machine?"

"Yes."

She gave me a web address to download a form I needed and said, "Fill out that form and fax it to me. It is Friday so we won't have time today, but we will work on getting this approved the first of the week. Also, send me a copy of the denial letter from Medicaid."

I thanked her and hung up the phone. I leaned back in my chair with my hands behind my head, propped my feet up on the desk, looked at Linda and said, "Problem solved."

It's a strange thing, I thought. Being self employed, I have a benefit that allows me to buy health insurance through the state government at a reasonable cost. One government entity says they won't help us anymore and the other takes over. Are they not part of the same government? I was glad I had kept this insurance active and they took Linda back on so easy.

I leaned back in my chair feeling good about what I had done. I fixed this problem. I took control. I knew what to do, and I was gloating about what I did. But the next week I would learn another lesson.

The following week we got the approval for Linda to be covered. Preexisting made no difference, but the coverage would not start for *two more months*. We still had more chemo and more tests, and it was expensive. What went wrong was I took control. God says to ask for anything and you will receive it (John 14:14). Jesus also said if two of you agree it will be done for you (Matt. 18:19).

I failed to ask God and decided to do it all under my own power. I know God sometimes answers differently than I might have imagined. I know His time frame is different from mine. I know He protects me by not giving me something I think I need, but I didn't even bother to talk to God. I took control myself, taking God for granted. He had been taking care of us and still does, but I decided what to do instead of turning the problem over to God. I didn't even ask Him for His blessing.

God can do more than we ask (Eph. 3:20), and I can do nothing on my own. But we must also ask for what is in His will to do for us (1 John 5:14).

Here we were about to enter into a two-month period with no insurance and no knowledge of the expense that lies ahead. It was time to trust fully in our Lord Jesus (Heb. 13:6). And that is not just for the rough times, but for every day of our lives.

Satan had tried to make us stumble with cancer, and he returned to try again. We finished out that month of insurance and the fifth chemo treatment. What lies ahead is one to three more chemo treatments and other unknown tests. We would have no active insurance for Linda at that time and no plans, but somehow, we knew and trusted that God had a plan.

We don't always choose the correct path God has for us. But He is always there to help us get back on the right path again.

SATAN CONTINUES THE ATTACK

Linda came home from the Cancer Center after her sixth and final treatment. Our church helped us pay for this one. Back when we learned of the cancer almost a year and a half ago, our church took up a collection to help us because we were uninsured. Because we did get Medicaid, we didn't use much of that money. After the cancer was beaten, and we felt like we were a safe distance past it, we began searching for other ways for our church to use that money. When we found out cancer had come back, I asked them to hold that money again. It was time for us to use some of the money our friends and supporters from our church gave to us. It is hard for me to ask for help, and I know it is hard for many people, but there is nothing better than having help around when you need it.

We did manage to get the price of the chemo treatments down from five thousand dollars to seven hundred dollars. Either they are not charging fair prices all the time or God was with us.

We were sure this would be the last treatment. She had six treatments the first round of cancer. Why should this time be any different? The doctor told her she would need to follow up this chemo treatment with another CAT scan so he could make sure the tumors were gone.

I called the hospital where the CAT scan would be done because Linda was still without active insurance. The person I talked to was Brenda. I remembered a Brenda after the day of surgery and things did not go so well with her. *We don't need another Brenda,* I thought.

I told Brenda our insurance had been canceled, and I was not getting much work so we were having a few money problems. They took off twenty percent for that reason, but the total cost was still over six thousand dollars.

We didn't have that much money and even the payments she offered would be more than we could handle. She said we might be able to get some help if we would bring in some more information on Monday.

I gathered all that she asked for. Most everything was already in a cloth bag we kept ready to go. Everyone wanted to see the same papers so they would know our income. We took it all to her on Monday, and she made copies and said she would call us in a few days.

Linda and I left Brenda's office, and we didn't talk much. Thoughts of no insurance, more tests, maybe more chemo, and no work were enough to keep our minds busy. *Didn't we already do this last year?* I once again thought about the book of Job and how he feared for the worst instead of trusting in God (Job 3:25-26). I thought about how easy it is for Satan to place a wrong thought and a lie into our heads. I decided it was time to stop the worry and time to trust in Jesus

Christ. I also thought about how hard it is to change the way we think.

A chemo treatment almost always creates about three depression days. We had started calling them chemo Sunday, Monday, and Tuesday. On this chemo Monday, Linda had one of her worst. She cried all day after we got home, and she felt worthless. I could do nothing. I was also fighting a little depression of my own. Everything seemed to be against us.

I had a lot of work quoted through five different customers at half off. Still the work hasn't come through. And half price work isn't much profit after expenses. What was God thinking? Many times I would ask God for work and get it the same day. Now it has been three months. Worry and depression were hovering over us.

Chemo Tuesday was not any better. Linda was feeling all the usual chemo side effects and I was of no help. Wednesday still held no answers for Friday's test. On Thursday, Linda called to see if they had any answers. We were concerned they would not do the CAT scan at all. They told her they had reviewed the case, and the test would be no charge.

Linda came to my office where I waste a lot of time when I have nothing to do. She told me the news from the hospital.

"That's great," I said without much concern.

I had enough on my mind that a free CAT scan didn't have much of an impact. I usually carry Linda through these chemo days, but this time I was down more than she was. I could only think about the next test or the chemo that might come after that. I tried to say the right things, but I know the positive sound was not there. I was carrying the same negative attitude that Job had.

"God is taking care of us," I would say. I did know He was, but I was not sure He was doing enough, and I didn't feel that He cared.

Linda left me alone in my thoughts, knowing she could do nothing when I was in one of my moods.

Linda did get her CAT scan that Friday, and two weeks later she went in for the results. I was still feeling a little beat up from life, but we knew she would only be there for a few hours. I stayed home to fix some broken furniture my kids had brought over. I knew the report would be just what we wanted to hear. I kept telling myself everything was fine, but in my heart, like Job, I was not so sure of it.

I had a late breakfast about nine o'clock. As I was eating, a tooth in the back of my mouth broke in half. It was a tooth that had a root canal about thirty years ago, so it had no feeling, but I knew it would have to be fixed. By twelve o'clock, I still had not heard from Linda so I called her cell phone.

"Where are you?" I asked.

"I am getting another chemo treatment," she said.

"Why?"

"I still have one tumor, but it is half as big as it was, so the doctor wants me to have another two to four treatments."

"Did you tell him he needs to put an extra week between them so the insurance can pay for it in September?"

"Yes, but he said the chemo treatments lose their effectiveness if they are spread out too far apart."

I was thinking about the money instead of my wife. Again I found worry of a different type trying to create stress. Money could be replaced; Linda could not. If I needed more money, I knew God would supply it.

I asked her, "Do you want me to come up there?"

"There's nothing you can do."

"Are you going to be all right?"

"I will be fine. I'll see you when I get home around five."

I hung up the phone and just sat there for about half an hour. Why is God allowing this to happen? I have no insurance and no work. This was our second battle with cancer and it shouldn't happen once to a Christian. Why does Linda need more treatments than she needed the first time?

I thought about how many times I have told others God doesn't give you these problems, Satan does. How many times have I said if you get everything you ask for, you would be God and God your servant, or sometimes the answers don't come as we might expect. It was my turn to feel confused. Where was God? Why wasn't He doing something? If I were a Christian of less maturity, I would be mad at God for allowing these things to happen. I would be blaming Him for the crisis. Not one time did Jesus ever tell someone He was going to make them sick to teach them a lesson.

"I just want to know what You're doing," I would say to Him. But no answer would come. "What am I supposed to do? What did I do wrong? What am I supposed to learn from this?" It was as if I was talking to myself.

I knew Linda would not be home until after five and it was about one o'clock. I decided to go for a drive. Sometimes I can hear from God when my mind is not so clouded with doubt and confusion. Driving helps my mind to not dwell on stupid thoughts, and I have had many conversations with God from my truck. In the past, I have even been mad at Him and yelled and screamed at Him. But I wasn't mad that day. I just wanted to know what was going on. What was He going to do?

I drove by our church on my way out, and I saw the minister's car in the parking lot. He was not going to have any words to help me today so I drove on by. I had not had lunch so I stopped for a cheeseburger. I hoped someone filled with the Spirit of the Lord might sit nearby and lift my spirit, although I was not sure anyone could say the perfect words that I needed at that time. I walked around the mall not even seeing the stores or the people. Everywhere I went for the day, I remained depressed and bewildered and empty.

I returned home a little before Linda. She just had treatment number seven, and number eight looked like a sure thing.

"Number seven is over. You have to have another one?" I asked.

"Yes."

"And after that?"

She said, "I will need another CAT scan to see if the last tumor is gone."

My first thought was, *that is after the other insurance kicks in*, but then I remembered we have not yet received Linda's insurance card. Nothing Linda had to say was restoring my confidence. I was, however, thankful her chemo was that day and this was not chemo Monday. I was not in a mood to help raise her spirit; I was still wrestling with my own and had been doing so for weeks now.

I spent the next few days feeling down also. Did I do something wrong? That can't be the problem. My sins are forgiven, and my works can do nothing. Am I not doing enough? God said we are to rule over the earth and subdue it (Gen. 1:28). He said we are to say to our mountains in life to move (Matt. 17:20). He said *you* resist the devil (James 4:7), and *you* lay hands on the sick (Mark 16:18). God has given us a way to live, and I follow the best I can in my understanding of His word, but was I to subdue the mountain with my words or turn it all over to Christ? If my words have power, it is because God put the power there. I can only do as He says to do; the rest is for Him. I can lay hands on the sick as God said, but He still does the healing.

The rest of the week passed, Sunday arrived, and it was time for me to give the next lesson at church. I usually have my lesson plans about four weeks in advance. Today was no different, but as I talked to God as I do before each class, I asked Him how I could teach when I don't understand our own problems at this time? It's funny how I know what to tell others as they face the problems in their lives, but the same problem in my own life seems so much bigger.

Once class had begun, the Spirit of God took over. His Spirit is always present in our class and somehow takes control. Sometimes, I don't have to teach, the natural flow of the conversation works under His power. Even in my distress I could tell God was with me (Heb. 13:5). I did notice, however, that the broken tooth was starting to hurt a little more.

After church, we went out to lunch. We always do this on Sundays. I could have skipped lunch that day because the pain from my broken tooth was growing. Linda and I often give thanks for our meals in silence. There are only so many ways to say thanks for the sandwich, so I do it in private, just me and God.

I don't mean to complain God, but don't we have enough problems? Why is this tooth hurting? Why can't I find a job? Why doesn't our mountain move, and why doesn't this cancer go away as I have told it to do? Oh yeah. Thanks for lunch. In Jesus's name, Amen.

That is not the best way to pray, but I was hurting. Jesus taught us how to pray in Matthew 6, but I am sure He understands my situation even if I don't.

We returned home, and I took a couple of aspirin. You know I am in great pain when I take more than one. I don't believe in covering up a sickness with so many chemicals you can't tell if it is gone or not. By five o'clock I had taken two more and it still got worse. At bedtime I took two more. Six aspirin usually last me for eight months. After tossing and turning until midnight, I went to sleep in another room so I wouldn't disturb Linda.

Finally, at two in the morning, I got up in so much pain I didn't know what to do, but I knew sleep was not going to happen with that much pain. I sat on the couch in the front room thinking of John 14:14.

Jesus, you said to ask for anything in your name and you would do it. Would you take this pain away and take this tooth away? Jesus you said to ask for anything. Ask for anything. These are your words Jesus. Ask for anything.

This went on for two hours as I rocked back and forth in pain with a pillow against my face. For two hours I said, "*You told me to ask for anything.*"

I have to admit, I wasn't feeling so sure He would help this quick, but after two hours the pain was gone. I was still swollen around the tooth. It should have been hurting, but it wasn't. I sat in that spot for another hour thanking God, and I thought the swelling was going down. It wasn't much, but I'm pretty sure it was going down. The pain was gone and I was amazed. I have seen God's blessings and wonders in my life many times, but I am still amazed with each one.

There have been many times in my life I wondered if God would help me. Before I had a relationship with Him, my own doubt and ignorance would stop up His blessings. The more I learn, the more I see Him giving. He gave to me that night, and I won't forget for a long time.

I went back to bed, and as I lay there, I realized I had been trying to do everything under my own power, not His. On my own I am nothing (John 15:5), but with Christ in me, all things are possible (Philippians 4:13). It is my faith that God was building upon. Yes

I wanted to know what He was doing. Who doesn't? But He wanted me to trust Him. Even when Israel was traveling across the wilderness, God gave them manna to eat for food for forty years. He gave it on a daily basis, and God wants my faith to be on a daily basis. The moment I try to walk without Christ, I will fail. As I was meditating on God's word, I fell asleep.

It doesn't matter if I go to bed early or stay up late, when the sun shines through the window, I get up. I told Linda about my night.

"I have to get this tooth pulled," I said. "I am not doing that again."

I called the dentist office that had taken out four other teeth of mine in the past five years. I was afraid I might have to take a drug to get rid of the swelling. I was also afraid they would not see me for a few days. My positive attitude was not that of a child of God, but at least for the moment, the pain was gone.

"Can you be here at two this afternoon?"

"Yes! I will be there."

"Bring someone with you to drive you home."

I hung up the phone. "I can't believe it," I told Linda in shock. "I'm going in today. I hope the swelling doesn't stop them from doing something."

I called my brother-in-law to be my driver. He arrived at my house about one o'clock. By two o'clock, not only was the pain still gone, but the swelling was too. The doctor said the tooth was beyond repair, and he would put me out and pull it. He had to put me out because the tooth roots were touching my sinuses, which made the operation dangerous. And I am a big baby in the dentist chair.

He pulled the tooth less than twelve hours after I was asking God to help and gave me pain pills that I never needed. Most importantly, my life was back on track trusting God on a daily basis instead of worrying about what God was going to do, or trying to do everything myself.

It is so easy to see what God has done. I need to quit trying to see what He is going to do. Now that my small problem was out of the way, I could focus on what God wanted me to do to help Linda. Thank you, Jesus.

Five weeks had passed. Linda had chemo treatments number seven and eight. The new insurance started on the first of September, and she had another CAT scan. It is so much easier with insurance. As Linda was getting the CAT scan and her weekly research test drugs, I was delivering a job to a new customer. I had been working the last three weeks, and it looked as if the new customer is going to provide much work.

We were both very excited. Linda was two weeks past the last chemo treatment, and there was a birthday party for two of our grandkids the next day. I made some money and found a new customer. Things were starting to look better.

We had not taken a vacation in three years. Some of the problems were results of the economy, but most of them were due to the cancer. Monday morning, we were going to a little cabin about two hundred miles from home. This two-night, three-day, mini vacation was given to us, and I believe it was a much needed blessing that God put together for us.

We would be in a secluded place about five hundred yards from a river and thirty miles from the nearest town. There was no television or telephone to distract us or remind us of the world. Even the cell phones would not work. We were going to forget about cancer, chemo, and the results of the latest CAT scan we would receive when we returned home. We had trails to walk and a canoe if we needed it. We could, if only for a few days, forget the troubles we have had and just see each other.

For a few days, we watched a nest of eagles, went on river walks, read our Bibles, and used the charcoal burner outside at least once a day. Every time we went outside, we had a dog that was almost always there to walk with us. The dog would happily take care of any leftovers and spent hours jumping, growling, and barking at any rock about the size of a turtle. It was so nice to forget about doctors and hospitals for a few days.

Seven years prior to this, we were on a vacation in the mountains. When we came home from that vacation, I opened the doors to my business, and we did so well that Linda quit her job to stay home and help me.

I like to think that this little vacation might just restart my business and recharge our spirit and our life. I don't know what abundant things God will place in our days ahead, but I know His plan is better than mine. We need only to trust Him as our children trust in us. He will supply all our needs (Luke 12:30-31). As Linda has told me many times, it was time to let go and let God.

THE HOLIDAYS

On our drive home from our vacation, I received a call on my cell phone from one of my older customers. He had a job for me to do if my price was still good. I had quoted the job eight months ago, and it was just now being released. I knew exactly which job it was, because I had always wondered why I didn't get it. I told him the price was still good, and I would start the job the next day. I thought about how God was getting things going before we even got home.

Chemo treatment number nine was also Thursday, but only if it was needed. Linda would go to the Cancer Center to find out if her cancer was gone, and I would go to work. We really did enjoy the few days off from the troubles of life, but it was also exciting to see what God was bringing to us in the weeks ahead.

I had been feeling down for a few weeks, and the time away from home did some good for both of us and recharged my faith. No matter what trouble comes into our life, God can make something good come from it, and we should always be thankful. Take the story of the ten lepers in Luke 17. They all asked to be healed, and Jesus did heal them all. After they learned they had been healed of leprosy, only one came back to say, "Thank you, Jesus" (Luke 17:16).

Jesus did ask, "Where are the other nine? Didn't I heal ten men?" (Luke 17:17)

All of our good gifts are received from God, and we should say, "Thank you, Jesus," giving glory to God for His grace and kindness. James 1:12-13 lets us know that life will provide trials and tests, and that no temptation is from God. Every good and perfect gift comes from God (James 1:17).

If we follow God and His ways, we will be blessed; if not, the door is open for Satan to easily enter. Take, for example, the commandment do not commit adultery. If you never do this you will never run the risk of getting a venereal disease or the other disasters that would come with this sin. Some of the things God asked us to do seem easy to understand . Others are easy for us to ask why. Instead of asking why, we should just trust in His all-knowing word and do it.

We have met people along this journey that had battled with cancer seven times. Some are taking dialysis five times a week. We have met people that have had transplants and loss of limbs. Do these problems come from not believing in God? No. They come from living in a fallen and sinful world.

Battling cancer has brought us closer to God, and I am sure Satan had a different plan in mind with this disease. We were not quite through with the discomfort yet, but we knew it was near the end. Whatever the outcome of Linda's test tomorrow, we will still be, as we always have been, in the hands of God. We are prepared to be finished with the cancer, and we have already given thanks (1 Thessalonians 5:18). We are fully trusting in the Lord Jesus Christ.

Many weeks passed and a small piece of the tumor lingered on. Chemo treatment nine took place, and ten had to be put on hold for one extra week because Linda's blood count was a little low.

Another CAT scan was taken after treatment ten, and it revealed the last tumor was still there but was very small and breaking up. Chemo treatments eleven and twelve had to be done. Treatment twelve was done on a Tuesday because our usual Thursday treatment fell on Thanksgiving Day. Linda had now had twice as many treatments this round as she did with the first round of cancer.

We have learned to wait on God. We may never know why cancer was being so difficult this time or what examples we may have been setting for others, but we knew the treatments and God were doing the right thing. God is never wrong.

It is often a little hard to see the blessings from God when they are still in progress. Cancer has taken us away from the path we would have walked if cancer didn't exist, but we know we will soon get back on that path. While we waited for the cancer to be gone, we had all grown to see how important each day is. I was working again, but not sixty or seventy hours a week. I could work the shorter work days and have more time to spend with loved ones.

Thanksgiving had always been at our house, and for the first time this year we went to our daughter's house. Linda just had her chemo treatment two days before, so the full force of the drugs had not yet kicked in and that kept her energy levels down. Thanksgiving was just as wonderful there as it would have been in our own home. All of our kids and all of our grandkids were there. And Linda did not have to do a thing except enjoy the kids and the day.

Thanksgiving is a day when two things take place: eating too much and being thankful for the life that God gave us. One look at my belly and anyone could tell I like to eat and don't really need a special day for that. Being thankful for life and the gifts from God are much more meaningful when you look around at your loved ones and know how important each one of them is. Not one of us will be around hundreds of years from now and no one knows the day or the hour that Jesus Christ will return, but it is a true joy knowing my family knows Christ (Mark 13:32).

December had arrived and another CAT scan was taken on the ninth day of the month. I had hoped Linda would have some of her own hair for Christmas. I knew it was not going to happen in only two weeks, but I felt the chemo must be over with by now. Linda usually felt good at two weeks after the chemo treatments, but this time, she seemed more tired. She'd had twice as many treatments this time, and I was sure that had some effect on her. We had also been shopping for

Christmas presents and perhaps that had added to her lack of strength.

Over the next few days, we did do some more shopping and were looking forward to the days our family would gather. That year, the plan had still not been settled where we would meet for Christmas. Our girls came over about two weeks before Christmas and spent the whole day helping Mom decorate the house. The grandkids had quite a time putting decorations on the tree as high as they could reach, and they all had to be lifted to the top to put something up high.

When Thursday arrived, Linda drove to the Cancer Center. It was time to see the doctor and get the CAT scan results. We were, as always, looking for a good report, but we are learning to go with the flow. Linda called me about ten in the morning with the report.

"The tumor is still there," she said.

"I didn't expect that," I said. "I guess you will be home late."

"No, I'll be home around noon."

"Are they not giving you chemo today?" I asked.

"No, my blood platelets are too low."

"That's why you have been so exhausted," I said. "Are they doing the chemo next week?"

"Yes, but I have to go to the hospital tomorrow and get a blood transfusion."

"Why? You have never done that before."

"They want to get my counts up so I can get chemo next week, and they said it would raise my energy level immediately."

"They want to give you chemo two days before Christmas?"

"No, they will be doing it on Tuesday. They will be closed Thursday."

We finished our conversation, and I felt like we were still being attacked. I worried Christmas would not be so good for Linda, because it would be four days after her treatment. She would be on her worst chemo days. I said a small prayer for her and went back to work. No sense in letting Satan cause more bad thinking.

Linda was worried about driving herself to the hospital Friday, so I took her in for her two o'clock appointment. They said it would take about three hours for the transfusion so I returned home. She called me at four o'clock, and I answered the phone.

"They are just now starting to put in the second unit of blood, so I will be here until at least six," she said.

"So, you were two quarts low."

"They're not quarts, but I didn't want you to drive over here and have to wait another hour."

"Okay, thanks. I will be over around six." I hung up the phone and headed out anyway. I thought it would be a good time to do some quick Christmas shopping. I forwarded the home phone to my cell phone so I would not miss any calls, and I went shopping.

I am not very good at Christmas shopping, and I didn't buy a thing. Here it is seven days until Christmas, and I still have nothing for Linda, but I was trying. I arrived in the room where Linda was receiving treatment about five minutes before six.

"Looks like a lot of blood still in that bag," I told her.

The nurse taking her blood pressure turned and looked at me saying, "It will be about one more hour."

I smiled at her and said, "I didn't know you work so late here."

"We work until nine o'clock," she said.

I looked at Linda. "I see they are putting in blood, but not taking any out."

"They don't take any out."

"I thought it was a transfusion, not an addition."

"They just call it a transfusion," she said.

"Do you feel better?" I asked.

"A little bit."

I sat down next to her and said, "Well, it is going to be after dark before they are done so it's good that I brought you in." Linda doesn't like to drive after dark.

There was a good side to all of this. Linda had the whole weekend to finish Christmas shopping and all the wrapping, and she would feel better with the new blood. The down side was, chemo would be on Tuesday, so she would not have a lot of energy for the Christmas weekend.

When Tuesday arrived, I took Linda in for her chemo treatment. I dropped her off and headed for a nearby town to visit with another new customer. At about noon, I had finished with the visit and was heading out for a quick lunch. Linda called me on my cell phone.

"You can come get me now," she said.

"It's not five o'clock. Are they not doing chemo?" I asked.

"No. They found another problem."

"What is it?" I asked as frustration formed in my mind.

"They found something growing in my mouth, and they don't know what it is, so they don't want to do chemo until they know."

"*They* are doctors, don't *they* know what it is."

"I have to go to a throat doctor to find out what it is."

"Okay," I said with disappointment, "I'm on my way."

The next few days, while we were waiting to get things set up for yet another doctor, I think my prayers were a little on the complaining side again. Every time we were close to being finished, another problem arrived. I was tired of the problems. But then I decided not to let Satan take charge of my thoughts again.

By Thursday, the usual chemo day, I was getting a little different outlook on this crisis, but Linda wasn't. It was only two days until Christmas, and I learned she had a different view of all of this than I was having.

Doctor Kevin was sending Linda to a throat specialist, and he used the word biopsy. That word biopsy put a new fear in Linda. She thought it must be a new cancer growing in a new spot.

"They do a biopsy to test for cancer," she said.

"I never thought of that," I said. "I don't see how you could possibly have any new cancer when they are treating you for cancer!"

"They are treating ovarian cancer. There are many other cancers they are not treating me for."

"So what? Many biopsies come back negative too. Let's not count this as something bad until we know if it is something bad," I said.

She was holding back her tears. "I just don't want any more problems," she said.

I took her in my arms. "I don't either. But look at it like this. Maybe it is a gift from God. You have now been five weeks without chemo making you stronger, and you got two units of blood making you feel better. That has never happened. And maybe God is doing something, so you will have a wonderful Christmas. Let's look at this as something good from God and put off any worry until we know for sure. You are always telling me to let go and let God."

"I do feel good right now," she said.

"And you will feel even better at Christmas," I said.

I know the fear of what might be didn't completely leave her. We always seem to think more of the worst instead of best.

Linda was trying to add more problems on top of the ones she already had. I can't honestly say I wasn't concerned, but I wasn't carrying the same alarm she was. We would find out sometime next week about what was going on, and I was okay with that, but the doctor's appointment time had still not been set.

It was still two days until Christmas, and I thought Linda might feel better if she got an early present. I handed her a package that was still in the plastic bag the store uses to package their sales. It had a large box inside, and I remember calling my daughter Leslie from the store the day I bought it to ask her if it would be a good gift.

"It's great!" Leslie said. "You can get me one if you want."

Linda took the package.

"Merry Christmas," I said. "How do you like my wrapping?"

"It's fine. You're a little early."

"I know. You just won't get anything else from me for Christmas, and I can't wait."

I got Linda a coffee machine that makes one cup at a time. There are over two hundred coffees that can be used. I like the smell of coffee sitting on the shelves at the grocery store, but I never drink the stuff. I was also a little unsure about buying a kitchen appliance, but this time it was what she wanted. It also gave her something else to think about and something else to do for the next few hours. She loves her coffee.

Christmas finally arrived. For so many years, Christmas would find the family at our house from six in the morning until late that night. Now that my kids had their own kids, things were changing. We went to Wendy's house that morning for a few hours to have a fantastic breakfast with her and the grandkids. We returned home around eleven to prepare for those coming to our house. By one o'clock our kids and grandkids arrived. Other family would be there about four-thirty.

Our grandkids came storming into the house. The tree was packed with presents, most of them for the grandkids, but they didn't even notice. They were filled with excitement, but not for themselves, their excitement was for me and Linda.

"Grandma, Grandpa! Open your presents," they were yelling as their mom and dad pushed them through the front door.

They were much more excited to see Grandma open what they had brought than they were about their own presents. The grandkids had to learn this from their mom and dad and God's church. It is better to give than to receive (Acts 20:35).

We opened one of our gifts the grandkids were shoving at us and then focused on the kids trashing the front room with wrapping paper for the next hour. It was a wonderful day. We all forgot about cancer, we forgot about the test coming up, and we forgot about the new doctor we were hoping to see next week.

We enjoyed our kids and our other company the rest of the day. We exchanged gifts and laughed and ate too much food. It was one awesome Christmas day for Linda, and she was feeling well.

Later that night, after all was cleaned up and the guests had all gone home, I sat in a chair across the room from our coffee table. On the shelf near the floor were four bird houses that were not there yesterday.

"Where did those come from?" I asked Linda.

"Wendy made them for me," she said.

They were amazing! Each one was different, and so many colors were used. Each one had a word on the front of it. The four little bird houses said *faith*, *hope*, *joy*, and *love*. I sat and stared at them thinking how wonderful our family was. I don't know if Wendy knows how much we are living on faith, hope, and love right now, but that day was full of joy. Somehow I felt better about Linda's new problems. I knew the joy of God was around us, and I knew He had a fantastic plan for us.

Our Christmas weekend was over, and Monday came around again. About nine in the morning, a call came in from the throat doctor's office. They told Linda her appointment would be for the next day at 3:30 p.m. The time was now set for the next worry to be settled in our walk with cancer. Did we have a new problem to add to the list, or could we ignore this one?

It wasn't long before they called back again to inform us that the insurance may not pay this bill because Linda was not referred to them by her primary doctor.

It is quite a game the insurance company plays. Doctor Kevin, who had been treating the cancer for over a year had to send us to Linda's primary doctor, so she could refer Linda to the next doctor. We had gone through this before, but this time, it was going on around a holiday week. Linda made a few more calls, trying to fix things to the satisfaction of the insurance company. It wasn't until the next morning, the day of the appointment that the throat doctor's office called with the okay to come on in, that the insurance requirements had been met.

We arrived a little early to fill out all the information required for a new patient. We waited in anticipation. I could see Linda was a little anxious.

"Stop worrying about what it might be. It might be nothing," I said.

"I'm just sick of being sick," she said.

I held her hand, and we sat there until she was called in.

We entered the room where the doctor would see us. It was a very big room with two of the walls filled with windows. We were on the third floor and the view was looking over a countryside spotted with houses. I could see a golf course about a half mile away. There was a chair for the patient that looked like it should be in the dentist office. Even the lights and other hardware connected to the chair looked like they too came from a dentist office.

In a short time, the doctor came in and greeted us. We exchanged the small talk as people do when they first meet. I really liked the man; he was very friendly, and you could tell he cared about us and our problem. We could also tell he was a man who knew Jesus Christ by the way he talked. We told him of the ongoing battle we were facing with cancer and chemo and the place in Linda's mouth that doctor Kevin was concerned with.

Linda had been worried about the biopsy and what they might find. She was afraid it might slow down her healing or add new problems on top of the problems we already had.

"I know how you feel," he said. "I have also had cancer."

That statement alone made us somehow feel better. He understood. He had been there. He looked healthy; he must have been healed. If he was healed of cancer, we could get through this too. Many thoughts flooded our minds as Linda and I would discover when we talked later.

"Sit up here in the chair, and let's have a look at what is going on," he said.

Linda took a seat in the chair. He picked up a flashlight tool with a funnel on the end and turned it on.

"Let's start with the easy stuff," he said. "I am just going to look in your ears and your nose."

He appeared to find nothing of interest and then asked Linda to open her mouth so he could see the real problem area. He looked at it for maybe three seconds.

"Okay," he said. "You won't need a biopsy on that, and it is nothing to be concerned with."

I think we both looked a little bewildered by his quick analysis.

He smiled and said, "This is a very common thing that happens to many people. This is the bone on the roof of your mouth, and they sometimes grow like this. Yours is as big as it will ever get, and you don't need a biopsy because it will never be cancer. The biggest problem this might cause will be if you ever need dentures. It might be a little harder to get them to fit."

"Will it go away?" Linda asked.

"No, and you probably didn't know you had it, did you?"

"No."

"It will never bother you or turn into cancer. You may have already had this for several years. I am surprised one of your other doctors has not talked to you about this."

"He's a gynecologist and he doesn't work on this end very much," Linda said.

The doctor laughed and sent us on our way with God's blessings.

On our way home, I told Linda, "He was a friendly doctor. I would change to this place if he wasn't a specialist."

"Yeah, so would I."

"I guess he will send a report to Doctor Kevin so you can continue chemo."

"I'm sure he will, but I will call them as soon as we get home."

"At least you had a good Christmas without chemo."

"And it is even better now knowing I don't have something else," she added.

Linda knew everyone at the Cancer Center, and when she called to give them the report, they set up her next chemo appointment for Wednesday of the next week. That gave her one more week without chemo, making it six weeks between treatments. It had given us a small glimpse of life without chemo. Her hair had grown out almost an eighth of an inch, and she had a small guide line for painting on some eyebrows. This would most likely be lost again, but the light at the end of the tunnel seemed a little brighter.

The New Year's weekend was next. We could not stay awake until midnight, so we called it a night about ten o'clock and went to bed. However, the midnight shotguns and fireworks woke us up. We laid there and talked until about one o'clock before we decided to get up and watch movies. We couldn't stay awake for midnight, but we watched the television until four.

We started off this New Year's Day much like all the new years before this one. We slept in and made no resolutions, because we have been around long enough to know we won't follow through, but we did pray for a better year than last year.

Most of us hope for a better year every year. We have never had one that stayed in our minds as a bad one, but this last year, so full of cancer, will likely be remembered for the rest of our lives. It will also be remembered as a year God carried us through many battles.

As for me, I have learned that one more day is a blessing from God. None of us has tomorrow guaranteed and each day has enough trouble of its own (Matthew 6:34). I give as much thanks for a new day as I do for a New Year. *Thank you Jesus for all the wonderful blessings you have given and for those yet to come.*

Linda went in for her first chemo treatment in the New Year, treatment thirteen, and we encountered another small dilemma.

"We have a small problem with your medication today," the nurse told Linda.

"What is it?" she asked as her heart raced with disappointment.

"Our freezer that has your test drugs in it has frozen over this morning and we had to reorder."

"Do I need to go home?" Linda asked.

"No. We can still give you the chemo treatment. We may be able to give you the placebo drug after it thaws out. I will ask the doctor."

They did have to reorder the drugs, and Linda had to come back two days later. The troubles of this New Year are starting out smaller than the troubles of last year. And the chemo amount was also cut back by 20 percent. Three weeks later, when Linda came in for her fourteenth treatment, her hair had not yet fallen out and was a quarter inch long. The cutback in the amount of drugs she was getting and six weeks of no treatments at all let her hair grow. We were still believing each week she was healed, and in three weeks, we would have the results from yet another CAT scan. We felt sure this test would verify that the last tumor was finally gone.

Whatever the results, we knew God was with us, today and always. "Thank you, Jesus."

WALKING IN GOD'S BLESSINGS

We had learned to find God's blessings in small and everyday packages. God wants us to live a rich and satisfying life (John 10:10 NLT), but we can only do it if He is in control. Yes, there are the big blessings that are coming, no cancer and eternal life, but we had to learn to look at what God had given us each day.

Another CAT scan was taken the second week of February, and we would soon hear the results. The weekly research test was still taking place, and we did not know for how much longer. This allowed the doctors to keep a closer eye on Linda, and we believed that too was somehow God's plan.

Linda's scar from the surgery was nearly gone. I thought a scar that big would never go away, but I know it was God putting us in the path of a doctor that knew what he was doing. I am still making breakfast most of the time, and I help Linda with most of the other meals. I used to leave all this in her hands, and I do still try to leave all the clean up for her. I dislike that part the most. But I have found cooking to sometimes be exciting to do.

Linda and I have found even with problems that life still goes on. We still have Thanksgiving; we still eat more than we should at Christmas; and another New Year's Day is still on its way. We have found we are more thankful each holiday because the whole family is together. We are thankful for the doctors we have had and the friends that helped support us. We are thankful Jesus walked with us and we are glad He is strong enough to carry us when needed.

The month of March had given us a few problems over the years. Linda had broken both legs, she had her appendix removed, and she received newfound knowledge of cancer, not once, but twice. This March is another one of the good ones. The chemo treatments were done and Linda has been off of the chemo treatments since January. They also pulled her off of the test drugs. She began receiving a very short treatment with a new drug every three weeks. For a while, Linda will spend about forty-five minutes a month at the doctor's office instead of twenty hours.

Linda's hair had begun to grow. It was too short to tell what it might do this time, but it was nice to see again. It appears to be about the same as last year, 60-percent gray. She felt a little apprehension about not taking chemo.

"When I was on chemo, I knew the cancer couldn't live. It feels strange not to be going in every week," Linda said.

"You felt strange when the kids moved out," I joked. "But you got over it pretty quickly."

We had reached another marker in our lives we will not soon forget. The battle with cancer lasted two years, and we won. We could look back and remember many times our Lord and Savior carried us and when He placed someone we needed in our path. Yes, we worried and wondered what He would do next, but God always took care of both of us.

A friend recently reminded me of a few of the miracles Linda and I had received the last few years. It caused me to remember more than a few, and I wondered if they were miracles or were they blessings.

A miracle, I thought, is an act of God—a supernatural event or a deviation from the natural laws that only God's almighty power can accomplish. Some of the blessings we had received were not far from that description. I thought, *If we are walking in God's blessings all the time, how could we ever need a miracle?*

I also remembered the greatest blessing (or miracle) of all. Jesus has made a way for us to get into heaven, and all our sins are forgiven . He did this for the whole world . He said He would forgive us and not remember our sins ever again. If we are without sin, why worry about judgment day ? If we are without sin, that makes us holy and blameless and without a single fault . This is a free gift from our Creator. Some will not accept this gift and some will choose to take their own way, thinking their way is better than God's way.

I remember two years ago on April 1, it didn't bring us laughter and jokes. It was the day of Linda's surgery to cut out the cancer. It was the beginning of a long and frightening battle. The battle was won and the cancer was gone. Unfortunately the cancer came back. April first last year, was the day of the first chemo treatment for our second battle with cancer. That battle was more than twice as long.

God has moved in amazing ways and given us many blessings in this walk with cancer. We have learned many things along the way. Even in bad times, Satan could not take us away from God, nor could he take God from us. Our bad times (though they were hard) only brought us closer to God. We learned to let go of many things that are not important, and not once did we do without something we needed. I had always hoped our journey through this crisis would help others fight some of their battles. I hope we have always set the correct Christian example and reflected Christ in our spirit. I hope we have shown no matter what the outcome might be with a crisis, Jesus Christ will always remain the only cure and the only way to heaven (John 14:6). I still need to be reminded once in a while to let go, and let God instead of trying to do it myself.

I can think of more than once with our cancer battle when it appeared so big and so hopeless that I wondered if God remembered us. Should I tear out parts of the Bible that appeared to not work for us? Sometimes I would see only the moment we were standing in and I wondered, *Where are you God? Why are you not helping us?*

I don't know why our battle has been so long, but in that time of doubt and confusion, in that time when I wanted to tear out scripture that didn't seem to work, I would look back at last week or last month. Sometimes it took me a while to see what God had already done.

Almost another year has passed. It is almost Christmas again. Linda started another round with chemo this past September. It's a different kind this time. It is five days a week every three weeks. Some of her hair has fallen out, but this chemo doesn't take all of it. The other emotional effects are also less with this type of treatment. We are both very tired of cancer. Her tumor is so small that chemo is the only option. The reports for the last five months have always been "It's a little smaller" or "It is not getting bigger."

Every Sunday our class room at church has prayer requests. There are often times when we hear of problems that seem overwhelming. In all the years I have been involved with our class, each and every person has had a very big worry or sickness pay them a visit. Linda is always reporting: "It is stable" or "Chemo starts again next week."

I did the closing prayer in our Sunday school class on the first Sunday of December. I walked to my wife and placed my hands on her shoulders and prayed with a lot of very long pauses as I tried to hold back the tears.

> Our Father in heaven,
>
> Each week we all have a prayer. Each week we give them to You. Each name on our list is important, but this week I want to pray for Linda. Father, we thank you for every gift we have received, but Father, we are tired of stable. Linda has been stable far too long. We are ready

> to get past stable and be healed. She is in Your hands where she has always been.
>
> In Jesus name.

It was a difficult prayer only being able to say a few words at a time, but I know God heard our request. I know God has not stopped giving to us. And I know God knows we have not lost our faith. Our battle has been longer than anyone would want, but we will not lose our faith or our hope or our love for God. If another battle comes, we will not give up. If Jesus needs to carry us some more, we will be ready. The battles are sometimes tough, but in the end, we know we will win.